Lecture Notes in Computational Vision and Biomechanics

Editors

João Manuel R.S. Tavares
R.M. Natal Jorge

Address:
Faculdade de Engenharia
Universidade do Porto
Rua Dr. Roberto Frias, s/n
4200-465 Porto
Portugal
tavares@fe.up.pt, rnatal@fe.up.pt

Editorial Advisory Board

For further volumes:
www.springer.com/series/8910

Lecture Notes in Computational Vision and Biomechanics
Volume 6

The research related to the analysis of living structures (Biomechanics) has been a source of recent research in several distinct areas of science, for example, Mathematics, Mechanical Engineering, Physics, Informatics, Medicine and Sport. However, for its successful achievement, numerous research topics should be considered, such as image processing and analysis, geometric and numerical modeling, biomechanics, experimental analysis, mechanobiology and enhanced visualization, and their application to real cases must be developed and more investigation is needed. Additionally, enhanced hardware solutions and less invasive devices are demanded.

On the other hand, Image Analysis (Computational Vision) is used for the extraction of high level information from static images or dynamic image sequences. Examples of applications involving image analysis can be the study of motion of structures from image sequences, shape reconstruction from images and medical diagnosis. As a multidisciplinary area, Computational Vision considers techniques and methods from other disciplines, such as Artificial Intelligence, Signal Processing, Mathematics, Physics and Informatics. Despite the many research projects in this area, more robust and efficient methods of Computational Imaging are still demanded in many application domains in Medicine, and their validation in real scenarios is matter of urgency.

These two important and predominant branches of Science are increasingly considered to be strongly connected and related. Hence, the main goal of the LNCV&B book series consists of the provision of a comprehensive forum for discussion on the current state-of-the-art in these fields by emphasizing their connection. The book series covers (but is not limited to):

- Applications of Computational Vision and Biomechanics
- Biometrics and Biomedical Pattern Analysis
- Cellular Imaging and Cellular Mechanics
- Clinical Biomechanics
- Computational Bioimaging and Visualization
- Computational Biology in Biomedical Imaging
- Development of Biomechanical Devices
- Device and Technique Development for Biomedical Imaging
- Digital Geometry Algorithms for Computational Vision and Visualization
- Experimental Biomechanics
- Gait & Posture Mechanics
- Multiscale Analysis in Biomechanics
- Neuromuscular Biomechanics
- Numerical Methods for Living Tissues
- Numerical Simulation
- Software Development on Computational Vision and Biomechanics
- Grid and High Performance Computing for Computational Vision and Biomechanics
- Image-based Geometric Modeling and Mesh Generation
- Image Processing and Analysis
- Image Processing and Visualization in Biofluids
- Image Understanding
- Material Models
- Mechanobiology
- Medical Image Analysis
- Molecular Mechanics
- Multi-modal Image Systems
- Multiscale Biosensors in Biomedical Imaging
- Multiscale Devices and Biomems for Biomedical Imaging
- Musculoskeletal Biomechanics
- Sport Biomechanics
- Virtual Reality in Biomechanics
- Vision Systems

M. Emre Celebi · Gerald Schaefer

Editors

Color Medical Image Analysis

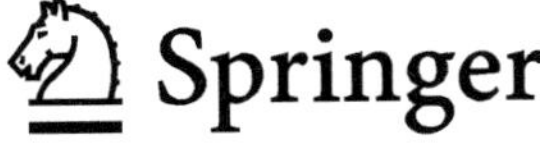 Springer

Editors
M. Emre Celebi
Computer Science Department
Louisiana State University Shreveport
Shreveport, USA

Gerald Schaefer
Department of Computer Science
Loughborough University
Loughborough, UK

ISSN 2212-9391   ISSN 2212-9413 (electronic)
Lecture Notes in Computational Vision and Biomechanics
ISBN 978-94-007-5388-4   ISBN 978-94-007-5389-1 (eBook)
DOI 10.1007/978-94-007-5389-1
Springer Dordrecht Heidelberg New York London

Library of Congress Control Number: 2012948955

Preface

Since the early 20th century, medical imaging has been dominated by monochrome imaging modalities such as x-ray, computed tomography, ultrasound, and magnetic resonance imaging. As a result, color information has been overlooked in medical image analysis applications. Recently, various medical imaging modalities that involve color information have been introduced. These include cervicography, dermoscopy, fundus photography, gastrointestinal endoscopy, microscopy, and wound photography. However, in comparison to monochrome images, the analysis of color medical images is a relatively unexplored area. The multivariate nature of color image data presents new challenges for researchers and practitioners as conventional methods developed for monochrome images are often not directly applicable to multichannel images.

The goal of this volume is to summarize the state-of-the-art in the utilization of color information in medical image analysis and provide future directions for this exciting subfield of medical image analysis. The intended audience includes researchers and practicing clinicians, who are increasingly using digital analytic tools.

The volume opens with "A Data Driven Approach to Cervigram Image Analysis and Classification" by Kim and Huang. The authors describe an automated, data centric system for cervigram image analysis that utilizes color and texture features extracted from the regions of interest to classify unseen cases using a Support Vector Machine classifier trained on several thousand annotated images. The authors report a sensitivity of 75 % and a specificity of 76 % on a set of 2,000 images.

The volume continues with four chapters on skin lesion image analysis. In "Macroscopic Pigmented Skin Lesion Segmentation and Its Influence on Lesion Classification and Diagnosis," Cavalcanti and Scharcanski investigate the influence of segmentation accuracy on skin lesion classification. The images are first enhanced using a novel shading attenuation algorithm. Following a segmentation step, various shape, color, and texture related features are then extracted from the lesions. Finally, the images are classified using a 1-Nearest Neighbor (1-NN) classifier. The authors compare six recent monochromatic and multichannel segmentation methods and conclude that the use of color information during segmentation improves the accuracy of classification.

In "Color and Spatial Features Integrated Normalized Distance for Density Based Border Detection in Dermoscopy Images," Kockara *et al.* propose an improved density based clustering algorithm for detecting lesion borders in dermoscopy images. This algorithm is an accelerated version of the celebrated DBSCAN (Density Based Spatial Clustering of Applications with Noise) algorithm and it does not require any preprocessing. The authors obtain promising results on a difficult set of 100 dermoscopy images.

In "A Color and Texture Based Hierarchical K-NN Approach to the Classification of Non-Melanoma Skin Lesions," Ballerini *et al.* describe a hierarchical classification system for non-melanoma skin lesions based on the K-NN classifier. The images are first segmented using a region-based active contour model. Color and texture related features are then extracted from the lesions. Finally, the images are classified using a hierarchical K-NN classifier. The authors obtain promising results on a set of 960 macroscopic images that contains five classes of non-melanoma skin lesions.

The final skin lesion analysis chapter, "Color Quantization of Dermoscopy Images Using the K-Means Clustering Algorithm" by Celebi *et al.*, investigates the applicability of a recently proposed k-means based color quantization method to dermoscopy images of skin lesions. This method improves upon conventional k-means based color quantization by using data reduction, sample weighting, accelerated nearest neighbor search, and deterministic cluster center initialization. The authors demonstrate that their method outperforms state-of-the-art quantization methods with respect to distortion minimization.

In "Grading the Severity of Diabetic Macular Edema Cases Based on Color Eye Fundus Images," Welfer *et al.* present an automated method for detecting and grading diabetic macular edema signs in color eye fundus images. First, the optic disc, fovea center, and exudates are detected using a sequence of morphological operators. The spatial distribution of the exudates around the macula center is then used to classify each case into one of four categories (absent, mild, moderate, and severe) using a CART (Classification and Regression Trees) classifier. The authors obtain an average accuracy of over 94 % on a set of 89 publicly available images.

In "Colour Image Analysis of Wireless Capsule Endoscopy Video: A Review," Fisher and Mackiewicz present a comprehensive survey of wireless capsule endoscopy video analysis focusing on the related color imaging aspects. After presenting an overview of the history of the field, the authors discuss feature extraction, segmentation, significant event detection, and adaptive control of viewing speed.

The volume continues with two chapters on microscopy. In "Automated Prototype Generation for Multi-Color Karyotyping," Wu *et al.* present a three-step method for generating a prototype from multicolor karyotypes obtained via multispectral imaging of human chromosomes. The first step involves the automated extraction of individual chromosomes from each karyotype, followed by chromosome straightening and size normalization. In the second step, the extracted and normalized chromosomes belonging to each of the 24 color classes are automatically assigned to a particular group based on the ploidy level. Finally in the third step, the prototype of the color karyotype is determined by generating a representative chromosome for each group using pixel-based fusion.

Bueno *et al.* in "Colour Model Analysis for Histopathology Image Processing" compare five color models, namely Red-Green-Blue (RGB), Hue-Saturation-Intensity (HSI), Cyan-Magenta-Yellow-Black (CMYK), CIELAB, and Hue-Saturation-Density (HSD), for the analysis of histological whole slide images. Based on visual examination and Receiver Operating Characteristic (ROC) curve analysis the authors conclude that the CIELAB model gives the best results.

A chapter on burn image analysis entitled "A Review on CAD Tools for Burn Diagnosis" by Sáez *et al.* completes the volume. The authors discuss the issue of color normalization and then present a comparison of several color segmentation methods applied to burn images. The chapter concludes with a discussion of color based estimation of burn depth using a Fuzzy-ARTMAP classifier.

As editors, we hope that this volume focused on analysis of color medical images will demonstrate the significant progress that has occurred in this field in recent years. We also hope that the developments reported in this volume will motivate further research in this exciting field.

M. Emre Celebi
Gerald Schaefer

Contents

A Data Driven Approach to Cervigram Image Analysis and Classification

Edward Kim and Xiaolei Huang

Abstract Cervical cancer is one of the leading causes of death for women worldwide. Early detection of cervical cancer is possible through regular screening; however, in developing countries, screening and treatment options are limited due to poor (or lack of) resources. Fortunately, low cost screening procedures utilizing visual inspection after the application of acetic acid in combination with low cost DNA tests to detect HPV infections have been shown to reduce the lifetime risk of cervical cancer by nearly 30 %. To assist in this procedure, we developed an automatic, data centric system for cervigram (photographs of the cervix) image analysis. In the first step of our algorithm, our system utilizes nearly a thousand annotated cervigram images to automatically locate a cervix region of interest. Next, by utilizing both color and texture features extracted from the cervix region of interest on several thousand cervigrams, we show that our system is able to perform a binary classification of disease grading on cervigram images with comparable accuracy to a trained expert. Finally, we analyze and report the effect that the color and texture features have on our end classification result.

1 Introduction

Cervical cancer afflicts an estimated 12,200 women in the US [1] and 529,800 women worldwide [2] every year. Fortunately, it can be cured if it is detected during its early stages and treated appropriately. However, among the new cervical cancer cases found worldwide each year, 85 % of them are in developing countries [2]. This disproportionate burden in low-resource world areas with medically underserved populations is mainly due to the lack of screening. Screening can prevent cervical cancer by detecting Cervical Intraepithelial Neoplasia (CIN), also known as cervical dysplasia. The CIN classification is specified in several grades: CIN1 (mild),

E. Kim (✉) · X. Huang
Department of Computer Science and Engineering, Lehigh University, Bethlehem, PA, USA
e-mail: edk208@lehigh.edu

X. Huang
e-mail: xih206@lehigh.edu

M.E. Celebi, G. Schaefer (eds.), *Color Medical Image Analysis*,
Lecture Notes in Computational Vision and Biomechanics 6,
DOI 10.1007/978-94-007-5389-1_1, © Springer Science+Business Media Dordrecht 2013

CIN2 (moderate), and CIN3 (severe). In a clinical setting, one of the most important goals of screening for cervical cancer is the differentiation of *normal/CIN1* from *CIN2/3+*. If a lesion is classified as *CIN2/3+*, it will require treatment whereas mild dysplasia in CIN1 typically will be cleared by immune response in a year or so, and thus can be observed or treated more conservatively.

To address the problem of CIN classification, we utilize a low cost, photographic screening test, called Cervicography. The photographs of the cervix, or cervigrams, can provide valuable and insightful information to assist in diagnosis and disease grading. One of the most important observations in cervigrams is the acetowhite region which is caused by the whitening of potentially malignant regions of the cervix epithelium after applying dilute (3–5 %) acetic acid. All forms of precancerous tissue exhibit some degree of opacity, or acetowhiteness, after contact with acetic acid. Thus, accurately interpreting the severity of this tissue region is critically important to cervigram image analysis. Additionally, other visual features or observations can assist with disease classification. These features include the identification or presence of mosaicism, punctation, atypical vessels or vasculature, blood, polyps, cyst, etc. However, as cervigram regions have very high variability in color, shape, and size, it is difficult for both trained medical professionals and computer algorithms to identify and characterize these regions individually.

2 Related Work

In recent years, there have been several automatic or semi-automatic image analysis algorithms applied to cervigram images. A common process in many of these previous works was the automatic detection of the cervix region. This region of interest (ROI) contains the relevant information necessary for accurate tissue and disease classification. In Li et al. [13], the region of interest is found by the analysis of local color features and optimized through expectation maximization. Zimmerman et al. [18] developed a two-stage segmentation process utilizing image intensity, saturation, and gradient information and reported their results on 120 images. Gordon et al. [9] uses a Gaussian mixture model to automatically find the cervix region of interest, and then separates the cervix tissue region into three types: the columnar epithelium, the squamous epithelium, and the acetowhite region. Gordon et al. also tested on a set of 120 cervigram images. Xue et al. [17] focuses on the removal of specular regions and the identification of the acetowhite region in the ROI. Similarly, Xue et al. tested on 120 cervigram images, and used $L^*a^*b^*$ color features, Gaussian mixture models, and k-means clustering to achieve their results.

Further image classification tasks in the region of interest can be performed as exhibited in several previous works. In Ji et al. [11], the authors use texture features to recognize important vascular patterns found in cervix images. They collected 5 images per vascular pattern class (network, hairpin, punctation1, punctation2, mosaic1, mosaic2) for a total of 30 images. Similarly, Srinivasan et al. [16] uses a filter bank of texture models for recognizing punctation and mosaicism on ten images.

As demonstrated by the previous work, there are many complex visual features that contribute to the problem of cervigram image analysis. The isolation of the cervix region of interest is an important first step used to remove the unwanted effects of the background image noise. Then, analysis of the region of interest can be performed by looking at color and texture features. Color features play a key role in the cervix and tissue classification task, whereas texture also plays an important role in the identification of mosaicism and vessel pattern analysis. Further, given the high variability exhibited by cervigrams, testing on larger datasets is necessary to validate the effectiveness of cervigram image analysis on real world datasets.

3 Methodology

In our work, we develop a unique approach to cervigram image analysis. In contrast to many previous works that utilize a more generative model towards cervigram image analysis, we developed a discriminative, data centric system that would be able to utilize similar cervigram cases in a collection of annotated cervigrams to perform a binary classification, i.e. *normal/CIN1* and *CIN2/3+*.

To be more explicit, we do not attempt to directly characterize the visual properties present in cervigram images. Instead, we utilize thousands of training images collected by the National Cancer Institute (NCI) and National Library of Medicine (NLM) to classify a new cervigram image. For this process, we will be utilizing two distinct databases. The first database consists of 939 expertly labeled cervigrams. There are detailed annotations linking these images to expert markings including the delineation of the cervix region of interest. We will refer to this database as D^1. Our second database, D^2, is of a larger scale and contains tens of thousands of patient records and cervigram images [10]. Each record also has been labeled with a final outcome, which we can utilize in the classification stage of our system. The final outcome is determined by expert practitioners and has been given a final diagnosis (*normal/CIN1*, *CIN2/3+*). These expert annotations of final diagnosis are based on analyzing the histology of the patient images, a commonly used gold standard to define the ground truth diagnosis.

In summary, our system takes as input a new test cervigram image and uses large amounts of training data to reach a final disease classification. This classification result involves several steps. The first step is the translation of raw image data into a compact color and texture feature representation. Using our representation, we can then attempt to leverage our first database of annotated cervigrams to isolate the cervix region of interest. Finally, we can again utilize our second database and the specific visual features located in the ROI of a given cervix region to obtain a final disease classification. By using the databases in our classification task, we are indirectly utilizing the variables that went into the diagnosis of a patient cervigram image, without having to individually model the complex visual characteristics.

3.1 Visual Feature Extraction and Representation

Through our research, and as exhibited in many previous works, we have found that both color and texture features are necessary to represent the visual cues present in cervigram tissue regions (acetowhite regions, mosaicism, punctation, etc.). Additionally, the relative size and position of abnormal characteristics are also important to capture in our feature representation. Thus, we utilize a spatial pyramid of color and texture features as described in Lazebnik et al. [12]. This spatial pyramid representation is able to preserve the geometric correspondence of visual features.

Color Features   Color plays an important role in cervical lesion identification and classification. One of the most important visual features on the cervix that have relevant diagnostic properties is the presence of acetowhite regions, or the whitening of potentially malignant cervical regions with the application of dilute acetic acid. The perceived color and thickness of an acetowhite region is also relevant to cervical lesion grading. Thus, we extract pyramid color histogram features, PLAB, from a cervigram image to represent various color regions. We convert the pixel colors in a cervigram into the perceptually uniform $L^*a^*b^*$ color space. A property of this color space is that a small change in the color value corresponds to about the same small change in visual appearance. Our PLAB descriptor is also able to represent local image color and its spatial layout. For each channel (L^*, a^*, or b^*) of the color space, we extract 3 pyramid levels, with a 16 bin histogram from each region. A pyramid is constructed by splitting the image into rectangular regions, increasing the number of regions at each level. Thus, a single channel histogram consists of 336 bins, and our complete PLAB descriptor consists of 1008 bins.

Texture Features   Texture features play an important role in representing various vasculature patterns, punctation, mosaicism, and tissue thickness characteristics. Similar to our color features, we represent texture as a pyramid histogram of oriented gradients, or PHOG feature [4]. The PHOG descriptor represents local image shape and its spatial layout. The shape correspondence between two images can be measured by the distance between their PHOG descriptors using a spatial pyramid kernel. To extract the PHOG descriptors from a cervigram image, we first compute the gradient response using a sobel edge filter. If we use an 8 bin orientation histogram over 4 levels, the total vector size of our PHOG descriptor for each image is 680 bins. For an illustration of our PLAB and PHOG feature, see Fig. 1.

Image Similarity Measurement   To compute the image similarity, we use a weighted sum of the similarities between the two images' color and texture features. The cost function that measures this dissimilarity, or distance, is defined as,

$$C_s(X, Y) = \lambda\big(d\big(X^c, Y^c\big)\big) + (1 - \lambda)\big(d\big(X^t, Y^t\big)\big) \tag{1}$$

where X, Y represent two distinct images, X^c, Y^c are the PLAB color feature vectors of X and Y, and X^t, Y^t are the PHOG texture features of X and Y respectively.

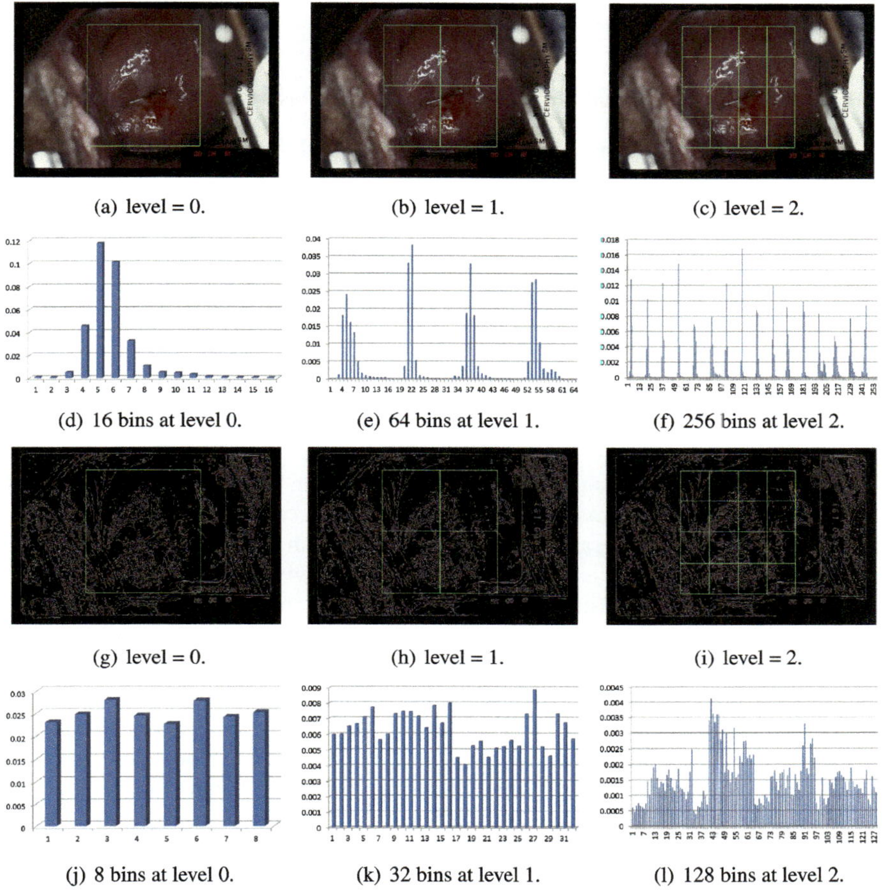

(a) level = 0.

(b) level = 1.

(c) level = 2.

(d) 16 bins at level 0.

(e) 64 bins at level 1.

(f) 256 bins at level 2.

(g) level = 0.

(h) level = 1.

(i) level = 2.

(j) 8 bins at level 0.

(k) 32 bins at level 1.

(l) 128 bins at level 2.

Fig. 1 Example of the PLAB and PHOG features extracted at multiple levels in a rectangular region of interest. In (**a**)–(**c**) the $L^*a^*b^*$ color space is sampled into 16 bins per region (per channel). The L^* channel in the PLAB feature vector is represented in (**d**)–(**f**). The edges of the input image are computed by a sobel edge filter and partitioned into a pyramid of regions (**g**)–(**i**). 8 orientation bins are extracted from each rectangle and concatenated into the PHOG feature vector represented in (**j**)–(**l**)

The distance between feature vectors is computed by d, and the λ term weighs the influence of the two features on the final similarity computation.

For the distance measure between two histogram-like feature vectors, h_X and h_Y, we use the χ^2 measure defined as,

$$d(h_X, h_Y) = \chi^2(h_X, h_Y) = \frac{1}{2} \sum_{k=1}^{K} \frac{[h_X(k) - h_Y(k)]^2}{h_X(k) + h_Y(k)} \tag{2}$$

where K is the total number of bins present in the feature vectors.

3.2 Finding the Region of Interest

In the first step of our algorithm, we isolate the (cervix) region of interest in a new cervigram. Given a new cervigram image our goal is to annotate a tight bounding box around the cervix. Some previous works have used the local color and position features in order to isolate the cervix region [8, 9, 17]. However, due to the high variability in color, size, and position of the cervix in cervigrams, these approaches based solely on local image features suffer from low specificity. In contrast, we take a different approach to the region of interest detection problem. Our approach is data driven; we rely on an expertly labeled database of 939 cervigram images with their delineated rectangular regions of interest in order to find a suitable bounding box for the region of interest in a new cervigram image.

We will refer to this step in our algorithm as our **optimized bounding box** method, and is defined as the following. Given a new cervigram test image, we extract the color and texture features from the whole image and compute the image similarity between this image and every other image in our 939 database (D^1) by Eq. (1). We sort the list of images in the database by decreasing similarity and extract the top M matching cervigram images. These images should *globally* resemble the test image; however, there is no guarantee that the cervix region of the top images match the location and size of the test image. Thus, we only use the top M matching cervigrams for their annotated ROI and use these ROIs as candidate bounding boxes. We denote the top M matching cervigrams' ROIs as B_m where $m = [1 \dots M]$, and our ground truth bounding boxes in D^1 as D_n^1, where $n = [1 \dots N]$. Then, for every candidate bounding box, we recompute the color and texture features of the test image inside the candidate ROI. We then compute the similarity between each candidate bounding box and every ground truth cervix ROI in our first database of N (=939) images. Among the $M \times N$ comparisons, we find the pair of ROIs that gives the smallest distance, and the candidate ROI in this pair will be our final ROI for the test image.

Mathematically speaking, we choose the minimum distance bounding box pair to obtain our final ROI, $\hat{B}_m$,

$$\langle \hat{B}_m, \hat{D}_n^1 \rangle = \arg\min_{\langle B_m, D_n^1 \rangle} C_s \left(D_n^1, B_m \right), \quad n \in [1 \dots N], \; m \in [1 \dots M] \tag{3}$$

3.3 Cervigram Classification

Given the cervix region of interest, we can now more accurately match a test cervix region to our database of cervigram ROIs. Our second database, D^2, consists of thousands of cervigrams that have been analyzed by experts and given a disease diagnosis of CIN1 through CIN3. This data can be utilized to train a classifier which will compute a disease classification for the given test image.

We build two classification methods into our system, a support vector machine classification and a majority vote classification.

3.4 Support Vector Machine Classification

In D^2, we compute the ROIs for every image, and extract their color and texture features. We then build a binary linear classifier that can discriminate between *normal/CIN1* and *CIN2/3+* using a Support Vector Machine (SVM) [5]. We extract our color and texture features from the cervix ROI and concatenate these vectors into a single 1688 bin vector (1008 bin color vector + 680 texture vector). We can build a SVM model based upon a subset of D^2, which will attempt to separate the two classes (*normal/CIN1* and *CIN2/3+*) in a high dimensional space. Given a new cervigram ROI, the SVM model can predict a CIN classification based upon the decision boundary obtained by our training data. We describe the size of our training and test set, as well as the parameters of our SVM model, and how we obtained them in our results section.

3.5 Majority Vote Classification

For our majority vote classifier, we again compute the extracted color and texture features in the cervix ROI. We can then compute a matching score between the test cervix ROI and every other ROI in our second database. Using the matching score, we can sort the similarity of the images to the new image and find the top Q most similar cases. These top cases vote on a classification, where the majority vote label is selected as the final output of our system. Mathematically speaking, given Q, the top cluster of $|L| = Q$ cases can be obtained by minimizing,

$$C(X) = \sum_{n=1}^{Q} C_s\left(\hat{D}_{L_n}^2, \hat{B}_X\right), \quad L \subset D^2 \tag{4}$$

where $\hat{D}^2$ are the computed ROIs from our second database, and X is our test cervigram, and $\hat{B}_X$ is its corresponding ROI. When minimized, the set of L consists of the top Q matches from our second database. Each element of L has a corresponding binary label i.e. *normal/CIN1* or *CIN2/3+*, and will cast a vote for the final classification. The majority vote label is assigned to the test image, X.

4 Results

We perform several experiments to evaluate our system. Our first experiment measures how accurately we are able to isolate the cervix region of interest. Our second experiment measures the ability of our system to correctly classify a new cervigram image. Finally, our third experiment measures the effect that our color and texture features have on the final outcome.

4.1 Isolating the Region of Interest

In this experiment, we analyze how accurately we are able to detect the region of interest in a new cervigram image. This experiment tests on 450 cervigrams in D^1, but utilizes all of the 939 (minus the test cervigram, e.g. leave-one-out) expertly annotated bounding boxes to obtain the final result as described in Eq. (3). The majority of the images are of the same size and resolution; however, there still is a small amount of variability. Our feature representations are normalized to account for this variability.

To measure the accuracy of our region of interest calculation, we use the Jaccard similarity coefficient defined as, $J(A, \hat{B}) = \frac{|A \cap \hat{B}|}{|A \cup \hat{B}|}$ which measures the similarity of our bounding box calculation to the ground truth region of interest specified by a trained physician. In this equation we can view A as the ground truth cervix region bounding box, and $\hat{B}$ as the minimum bounding box found in Eq. (3). In essence, the Jaccard coefficient can be viewed as the area of intersection of bounding boxes, divided by the total area covered by both bounding boxes. A Jaccard similarity coefficient closer to one has a greater similarity to the ground truth; whereas, a coefficient value close to zero has nearly no overlap area similar to the ground truth. In this experiment, we compare three different methods.

1. **Image Bounding Box** (IBB). In this method, we choose the most similar image to the test image, based upon a global image similarity. The bounding box is transferred from the top match to the test cervigram. This method does not eliminate the noise present outside the region of interest.
2. **Average Bounding Box** (ABB). This method again uses global image similarity; however, we take the top K matches and average the position of their bounding boxes to achieve our final bounding box. We used a gradient descent on the Jaccard similarity coefficient (with respect to D^1) to obtain the best K ($= 15$).
3. **Optimized Bounding Box** (OBB). This is our method described in Sect. 3.2 that utilizes candidate bounding boxes from a global image match. We compute the final bounding box by finding the *argmin* in Eq. (3). For our experiments, we set M to be 100, i.e. we have 100 candidate bounding boxes to choose from.

We show several sample images, their corresponding ground truth bounding boxes, and the results of these three methods in Fig. 2.

However, the Jaccard index does not describe the entire story. As seen in Fig. 2(4)(c), the Jaccard index can be quite low, yet the cervix region may be more accurately located than indicated. To further describe the accuracy of our cervix ROI calculation, we compute the Euclidean distance between the ground truth centroid position, and our computed ROI centroid position. Additionally, we record the difference of the aspect ratio between the ground truth bounding box and our computed rectangle as further evidence. The aspect ratio is computed by the absolute difference between the width divided by height of the computed bounding box and the width divided by height of the ground truth bounding box. In Table 1 we report the average Jaccard index values, centroid difference, and aspect ratio difference. And

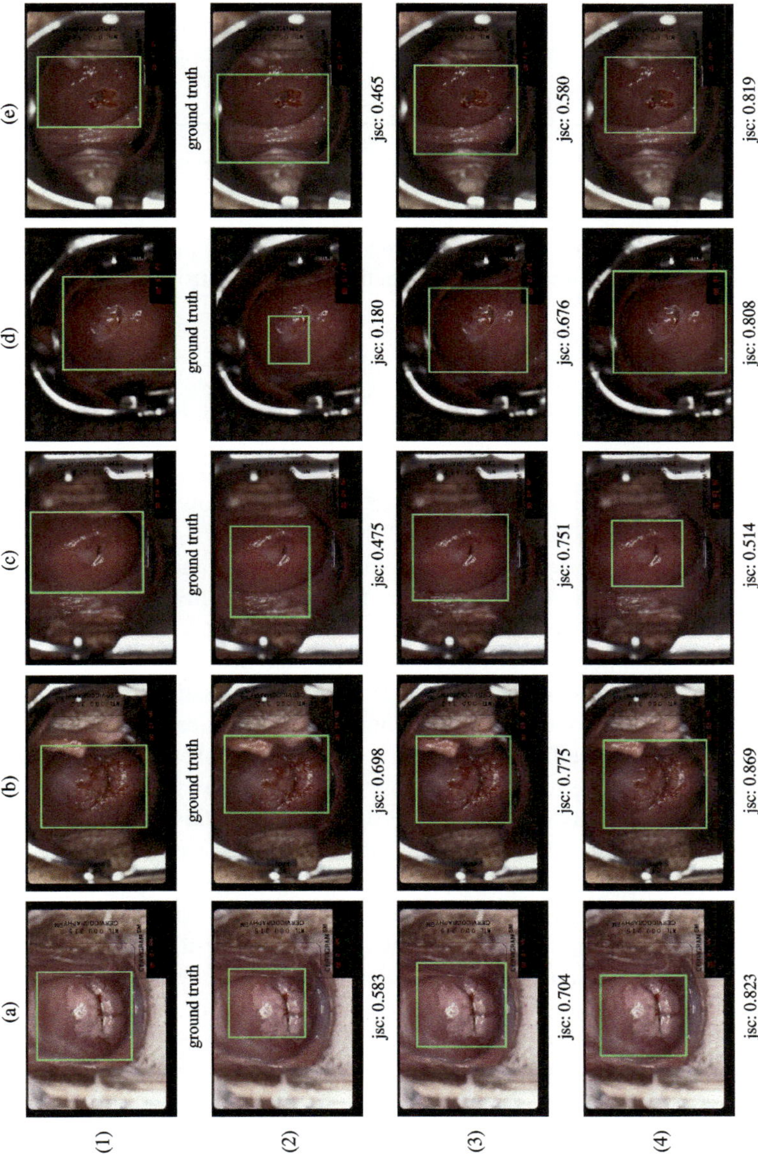

Fig. 2 Sample region of interest calculations on five (**a**)–(**e**) images. The ground truth (*1*) and expert annotations are shown here. The image bounding box (IBB) (*2*), average bounding box (ABB) (*3*), and optimized bounding box (OBB) (*4*) and their corresponding Jaccard (jsc) coefficients are also displayed. In *column* (*c*) *row* (*4*), we see a low Jaccard index, but visually close ROI calculation

Table 1 Comparison of three different region of interest methods. We report the average Jaccard index, centroid distance, and aspect ratio difference of the computed bounding box and ground truth bounding box on 450 test images

Method	Jaccard index (std)	Centroid dist.	Aspect ratio
Image Bounding Box (IBB)	0.611 (0.12)	32.37	0.148
Average Bounding Box (ABB)	0.699 (0.13)	23.91	0.109
Optimized Bounding Box (OBB)	0.736 (0.14)	25.72	0.096

std = Standard Deviation

as seen from our results, our optimized bounding box method outperforms the other two methods, and has the desired effect of maintaining a low centroid difference and consistent aspect ratio.

4.2 Accuracy of Our Disease Classification

In our second experiment, we utilize a subset of 2,000 cervigram images obtained from the NIH/NCI database D^2, consisting of 1,000 *normal/CIN1* grade images and 1,000 *CIN2/3+* cases. We perform a ten fold cross validation, binary classification on this dataset to evaluate how well our system is able to differentiate between these classes. We test using two classifiers, our majority vote classifier described in Sect. 3.5 and a linear Support Vector Machine described in Sect. 3.4.

There are several parameters that need to be set for both classification methods. For our majority vote technique, we train the number of voting cases, Q, by computing the Dice similarity coefficient, $DSC = \frac{2 \cdot TP}{(2 \cdot TP + FP + FN)}$ over our training set while varying Q between the top matching case ($Q = 1$) to the top fifty ($Q = 50$) matches. In the Dice similarity coefficient, TP denotes true positive cases, FP denotes false positive cases, and FN are false negative cases. As we increase Q, the DSC score steadily increases from 0.70 at $Q = 1$ and asymptotically approaches 0.75 when $Q > 30$. Therefore, we set Q to be the top 33 most similar cervigram images to the input image that will vote to obtain the final classification output of our system. For the weight parameter of our color versus texture features (λ value), we chose $\lambda = 0.7$. The analysis behind this value can be seen in the next section, Sect. 4.3.

For our linear SVM, we train the parameters of our model using a five-fold cross validation on the training images, and use this model to classify the new input image. The results of both our methods can be seen in Table 2. Additionally, in this table, we also report comparative results from multiple studies around the world as reported by Sankaranarayanan et al. [15]. In these studies, direct visual inspection of the cervix was conducted after the application of acetic acid, and each patient is given a result of positive or negative for *CIN2/3+*.

Table 2 Comparison of Sensitivity, and Specificity for different classification methods for detecting *CIN2/3+*. Our automatic classification method is comparable to manual inspection by experts

Method	Samples[a]	Sensitivity, % (95 % CI)	Specificity, % (95 % CI)
Our automatic method[b], Majority Vote	2,000	73 (65–81)	77 (67–87)
Our automatic method[b], L-SVM	2,000	75 (69–82)	76 (66–86)
Denny et al. [6], 2000, South Africa	2,885	67 (56–77)	84 (82–85)
Belinson et al. [3], 2001, China	1,997	71 (60–80)	74 (71–76)
Denny et al. [7], 2002, South Africa	2,754	70 (59–79)	79 (77–81)
Sankaranarayanan et al. [14], 2004 India and Africa	54,981	79 (77–81)	86 (85–86)

[a]Samples for our method are number of distinct cervigram images. Samples for the comparative studies correspond to number of patients

[b]Confidence intervals calculated by ten-fold cross validation

CI = Confidence Interval

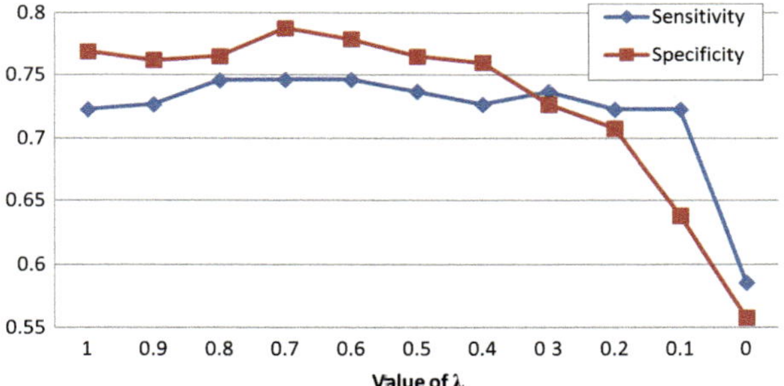

Fig. 3 The effect of changing our λ value between 1–0 when using a majority vote classifier. A balanced weight of 0.5 has equal contribution of color and texture, whereas a value closer to 1 favors the color feature. Empirically, a λ value of 0.7 has the best specificity and sensitivity on D^2

4.3 Weighted Effect of Color and Texture

In our final experiment, we view the effects of the color and texture features on our final classification result. Using our majority vote classifier, and altering the λ in Eq. (1), we can evaluate the influence of these features. As a baseline data point, a value of $\lambda = 0.5$, gives both color and texture features equal weight. On a set of 1,000 cervigram images from D^2 (500 *normal/CIN1*, 500 *CIN2/3+*), we vary the parameter from 0–1, where a λ of less than 0.5 gives more weight to our texture feature and a λ of greater than 0.5 gives more weight to our color feature. We analyze how this parameter affects the sensitivity and specificity of our majority vote classifier on dataset, D^2 and display the results in Fig. 3.

From these results it is clear that the color feature plays a vital role in the CIN designation for cervigram images. By using the color feature alone ($\lambda = 1$), we are still able to achieve fairly good results, but if we only use texture features ($\lambda = 0$), our sensitivity and specificity drop dramatically.

5 Discussion and Conclusion

We present an automatic cervigram image analysis algorithm that is able to isolate the region of interest in a new cervigram image, and ultimately classify the image as *normal/CIN1* or *CIN2/3+*. Our system is data centric, meaning we do not attempt to directly model the complex features present in the cervix anatomy, but rather utilize thousands of training images to perform our analysis. Furthermore, our system performs well, and is shown to be comparable to human observers. To improve our results, we have been exploring multi-modal classification methods by utilizing patient data such as patient age, HPV types (16/18/31), and health behavior (history of smoking). Another possible improvement would be the use of vector weights to find the optimal balance of color and texture. As a final note, since a color change of the acetowhite region has a high correlation to the severity of a CIN classification, this would suggest that a color feature would be important in cervigram image analysis. Through our experiments, we were able to confirm that color does in fact play a vital role in the CIN classification task.

Acknowledgements This research was supported in part by the Intramural Research Program of the National Institutes of Health (NIH), National Library of Medicine (NLM), and Lister Hill National Center for Biomedical Communications (LH- NCBC). The image and clinical data for this work comes from the National Cancer Institute (NCI) Guanacaste/ALTS projects.

References

1. Atlanta (2010) Cancer facts and figures. American Cancer Society, Atlanta
2. Atlanta (2011) Global cancer facts and figures, 2nd edn. American Cancer Society, Atlanta
3. Belinson J, Pretorius R (2002) Cervical cancer screening by simple visual inspection after acetic acid. Obstet Gynecol 99(3):518
4. Bosch A, Zisserman A, Munoz X (2007) Representing shape with a spatial pyramid kernel. In: International conference on image and video retrieval, pp 401–408
5. Chang CC, Lin C.J. (2001) LIBSVM: a library for support vector machines. Software available at http://www.csie.ntu.edu.tw/~cjlin/libsvm
6. Denny L, Kuhn L, Pollack A, Wainwright H, Wright T Jr (2000) Evaluation of alternative methods of cervical cancer screening for resource-poor settings. Cancer 89(4):826–833
7. Denny L, Kuhn L, Pollack A, Wright T Jr (2002) Direct visual inspection for cervical cancer screening. Cancer 94(6):1699–1707
8. Gordon S, Zimmerman G, Greenspan H (2004) Image segmentation of uterine cervix images for indexing in PACS. In: IEEE symposium on computer-based medical systems
9. Gordon S, Zimmerman G, Long R, Antani S, Jeronimo J, Greenspan H (2006) Content analysis of uterine cervix images: initial steps towards content based indexing and retrieval of cervigrams. In: Proceedings of SPIE medical imaging, vol 6144, pp 1549–1556
10. Jeronimo J, Long L, Neve L, Michael B, Antani S, Schiffman M (2006) Digital tools for collecting data from cervigrams for research and training in colposcopy. J Low Genit Tract Dis 10(1):16
11. Ji Q, Engel J, Craine E (2000) Classifying cervix tissue patterns with texture analysis. Pattern Recognit 33(9):1561–1574
12. Lazebnik S, Schmid C, Ponce J (2006) Beyond bags of features: spatial pyramid matching for recognizing natural scene categories. In: IEEE computer society conference on computer vision and pattern recognition, vol 2, pp 2169–2178

13. Li W, Gu J, Ferris D, Poirson A (2007) Automated image analysis of uterine cervical images. Prog Biomed Opt Imaging 8(33)
14. Sankaranarayanan R, Basu P, Wesley R, Mahe C, Keita N, Mbalawa C, Sharma R, Dolo A, Shastri S, Nacoulma M et al (2004) Accuracy of visual screening for cervical neoplasia: results from an IARC multicentre study in India and Africa. Int J Cancer 110(6):907–913
15. Sankaranarayanan R, Gaffikin L, Jacob M, Sellors J, Robles S (2005) A critical assessment of screening methods for cervical neoplasia. Int J Gynecol Obstet 89:S4–S12
16. Srinivasan Y, Nutter B, Mitra S, Phillips B, Sinzinger E (2006) Classification of cervix lesions using filter bank-based texture mode. In: IEEE symposium on computer-based medical systems
17. Xue Z, Antani S, Long R, Thoma G (2007) Comparative performance analysis of cervix roi extraction and specular reflection removal algorithms for uterine cervix image analysis. In: Proceedings of SPIE medical imaging, vol 6512, pp 4I1–4I9
18. Zimmerman-Moreno G, Greenspan H (2006) Automatic detection of specular reflections in uterine cervix images. In: Proceedings of SPIE medical imaging

Macroscopic Pigmented Skin Lesion Segmentation and Its Influence on Lesion Classification and Diagnosis

Pablo G. Cavalcanti and Jacob Scharcanski

Abstract Melanoma is a type of malignant pigmented skin lesion, and currently is among the most dangerous existing cancers. However, differentiating malignant and benign cases is a hard task even for experienced specialists, and a computer-aided diagnosis system can be an useful tool. Usually, the system starts by pre-processing the image, i.e. removing undesired artifacts such as hair, freckles or shading effects. Next, the system performs a segmentation step to identify the lesion boundaries. Finally, based on the image area identified as lesion, several features are computed and a classification is provided. In this chapter we describe all these steps, giving special attention to segmentation approaches for pigmented skin lesions, proposed for standard camera images (i.e. simple color photographs). Next, we compare the segmentation results to identify which techniques have more accurate results, and discuss how these results may influence in the following steps: the feature extraction and the final lesion classification.

1 Introduction

Pigmented skin lesions include both, benign and malignant forms. According to World Health Organization [1], about 132000 melanoma cases, a dangerous kind of malignant pigmented skin lesion, occur globally each year. The early diagnosis of melanomas is very important for the patient prognosis, since most malignant skin lesion cases can be treated successfully in their early stages. However, research work has shown that discriminating benign from malignant skin lesions is a challenging task [2, 3].

To help diagnosing pigmented skin lesions, physicians often use dermoscopy, which is a non-invasive technique that magnifies submacroscopic structures with

P.G. Cavalcanti (✉) · J. Scharcanski
Instituto de Informática, UFRGS, Av. Bento Gonçalves 9500, Porto Alegre, Brazil
e-mail: pgcavalcanti@inf.ufrgs.br

J. Scharcanski
e-mail: jacobs@inf.ufrgs.br

M.E. Celebi, G. Schaefer (eds.), *Color Medical Image Analysis*,
Lecture Notes in Computational Vision and Biomechanics 6,
DOI 10.1007/978-94-007-5389-1_2, © Springer Science+Business Media Dordrecht 2013

the help of an optical lens (a dermoscope) and liquid immersion. According to Mayer [4], the use of dermoscopy can increase the diagnosis sensitivity in 10–27 % with respect to the clinical diagnosis. Also, several automatic segmentation and classification methods have been proposed to help obtain a diagnosis with a dermoscopy image [5–10]. However, even with the help of dermoscopy, differentiating malignant and benign lesions is a challenging task. In fact, specialists affirm that in the early evolution stages of malignant lesions, dermoscopy may not be helpful since it often does not improve the diagnosis accuracy [11].

Still considering early stage cases, there are practical situations where a non-specialist (e.g. a physician not trained on Dermatology) wishes to have a qualified opinion about a suspect skin lesion, but only standard camera imaging is available on site. In such situations, telemedicine is justifiable, and the non-specialist can capture a macroscopic pigmented skin lesion (MPSL) image of the suspect skin lesion and send it to a specialist, who can analyze it in higher detail. In this particular situation, a teledermatology consultation brings benefits, like the easier access to health care and faster clinical results [12]. Besides, comparing the physical (face-to-face) patient diagnosis with the remote diagnosis by teledermatology, recent results suggest that teledermatology also tends to be effective and reliable [13].

In the last decades, several segmentation techniques have been proposed to facilitate the remote diagnosis of MPSL images. Since there is no standardized protocol for acquiring these images, often they contain artifacts like hair, shading and other disturbances that make the remote diagnosis by specialists more difficult. With the help of the automatic segmentation, this task may be facilitated. Moreover, the segmentation is an initial step for computer-aided diagnosis systems. Starting from the lesion area identification, lesion features can be extracted and an automatic classification/diagnosis can be provided.

However, since these MPSL images may present characteristics that could make the remote diagnosis more difficult, the automatic processing and analysis also poses some challenges for the researchers in this field. Most of the MPSL image segmentation techniques proposed in the literature convert the original color image to a monochromatic image, and use a thresholding algorithm to identify the lesion area [14–17]. Even more complex segmentation approaches, such as active contours techniques [18, 19], process grayscale images. Nevertheless, the discriminating lesion and healthy skin areas may be more difficult on a monochromatic images, since the chromatic aspect is lacking in them.

In the following sections we will present segmentation algorithms that process multichannel MPSL images, based on thresholding [20] and on level-sets [21]. After that, we show that such methods working on multichannel MPSL images are more efficient than methods working on monochromatic images. Also, we will discuss how features that are relevant from the medical point of view can be extracted, and how the final classification/diagnosis of the acquired lesion is affected by the segmentation quality.

2 Pre-processing

MPSL images usually contain artifacts that make the segmentation process more difficult. Skin characteristics, such as freckles, are easily detected by these algorithms based on color or size. However, most methods available try to identify the lesion area assuming that pigmented skin lesions correspond to locally darker skin discolorations. Consequently, artifacts such as hair and shading, that usually also are darker than healthy skin may be mistaken as lesions during the segmentation process.

Although some of the approaches available eliminate hair as a pre-processing step [15, 16, 19], this task can be performed as a post-processing step, after the image segmentation. Hair is thin, and its shape is quite distinct from the lesion shapes, and consequently it is easy to eliminated hair from MPSL images by morphological operations or other methodologies.

On the other hand, the presence of shading requires pre-processing in advance to segmentation. The shading areas assume any shape, and require a treatment that is different from that given to artifacts like hair. Moreover, if the shading attenuation is well performed, it also contributes for the enhance the contrast between healthy and unhealthy skin.

2.1 Shading Attenuation

Alcón et al. [17] proposed to correct the uneven illumination by removing the low frequency spatial component of the image. Although this method can be efficient for some images, it requires specific parameters. It is very difficult to obtain a specific value that can be used for any input image, and the authors [17] do not detail how to obtain this value automatically.

Face images also are skin images and can be affected by shading effects. Tan and Triggs [22] and Zhou et al. [23] proposed to use Difference of Gaussians (DoG) filtering to correct the shading artifacts. However, this methodology needs specific parameters (e.g., definition of a window size and the filters standard deviations) which may require adjustments for different types of shading effects in the skin lesion images. Moreover, the authors observed that DoG filtering may generate strong-edges in hair areas [22], which could affect negatively the overall segmentation process.

Therefore, Cavalcanti et al. [21] proposed a shading attenuation method that is adaptive to the MPSL image data. Their method assumes that images are acquired in a way that the lesion appears in the image center, and it does not touch the image outer borders. The first step of the method is to convert the image from the original RGB color space to the HSV color space, and retain the Value channel V. This is justified by the fact that this channel presents the higher visibility of the shading effects. A region of 20×20 pixels is extracted from each V corner, and the union of these four sets define the pixel set S. This pixel set is used to adjust the following quadric function $z(x, y)$:

$$z(x, y) = P_1 x^2 + P_2 y^2 + P_3 xy + P_4 x + P_5 y + P_6, \tag{1}$$

Fig. 1 Shading attenuation example. (**a**) Input image; (**b**) Obtained quadric model using the corners of the input Value channel; (**c**) Obtained quadric model in 3D; (**d**) Result obtained by the division of the Value channel by the obtained quadric model

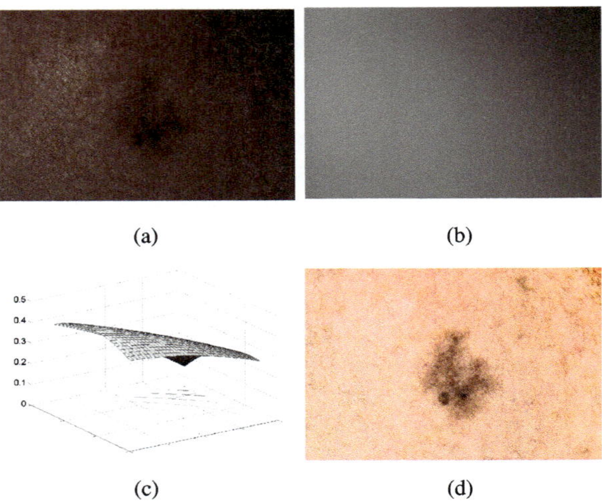

(a)

(b)

(c)

(d)

where the six quadric function parameters P_i ($i = 1, \ldots, 6$) are chosen to minimize the error ε:

$$\varepsilon = \sum_{j=1}^{N_s} \left[V(S_{j,x}, S_{j,y}) - z(S_{j,x}, S_{j,y}) \right]^2, \tag{2}$$

where, $S_{j,x}$ and $S_{j,y}$ are the x and y coordinates of the jth element of the set S, respectively, and N_s is the total number of pixels of the four corners (in our case, $N_s = 1600$).

Calculating the quadric function $z(x, y)$ for each image spatial location (x, y), we have an estimate $z(x, y)$ of the local illumination intensity in the image $V(x, y)$. Dividing the original $V(x, y)$ channel by $z(x, y)$, we obtain a new Value channel where the shading effects have been attenuated. The final step is to replace the original Value channel by this new Value channel, and convert the image from the HSV color space to the original RGB color space. In Fig. 1, an example of applying this method to a skin lesion image is presented. The result is a color image easier to be segmented.

3 Segmentation

As already mentioned in Sect. 1, several segmentation techniques have been proposed for MPSL images in the last decades. We outline some representative recent methods and their characteristics in the following subsections. Also, at the end of this section, we present and discuss the performance of these segmentation techniques for a MPSL image database.

3.1 Grayscale-Based Methods

Based on the principle that a pigmented skin lesion is a depigmentation of the skin, and to reduce the computation cost, many segmentation methods start by converting the input image from color to grayscale. After that, most algorithms try to distinguish between healthy to unhealthy pixels. The following techniques illustrate the algorithms that have recently been used for this purpose.

3.1.1 Thresholding-Based Methods

Otsu's Thresholding method [24] has been widely used in grayscale images [14–16]. Furthermore, Cavalcanti et al. [25] also employed this thresholding scheme to the Red channel (R of the RGB color space), trying to take advantage of the fact that healthy skin usually has a reddish tone. This method assumes two pixel classes, namely healthy and unhealthy skin pixels, and searches exhaustively for the threshold th that minimizes the total intra-class variance $\sigma_w^2(th)$, defined as the weighted sum of variances of the two classes:

$$\sigma_w^2(th) = \omega_1(th)\sigma_1^2(th) + \omega_2(th)\sigma_2^2(th), \tag{3}$$

where ω_i are the a priori probabilities of the two classes separated by the threshold th, and σ_i^2 are their intra-class variances. Minimizing the intra-class variance is equivalent to maximizing the inter-class variance $\sigma_b^2(th)$:

$$\begin{aligned}\sigma_b^2(th) &= \sigma^2 - \sigma_w^2(th) \\ &= \omega_1(th)\omega_2(th)\left[\mu_1(th) - \mu_2(th)\right]^2,\end{aligned} \tag{4}$$

where σ^2 is the image pixels variance, and μ_i are the class means. Computed the th threshold, the lesion pixels correspond to the pixels with values lower than th.

The Otsu's method usually is followed by a post-process step, constituted by successive morphological operations, to eliminate other regions that may be thresholded (besides the lesion). Cavalcanti et al. [25] suggest the following procedures: select the largest threshold area, perform a hole filling operation, and a dilation with a disk with 5 pixels of radius.

However, Alcón et al. [17] recently suggested that Otsu's method may over-segment the lesion area. So, they proposed a new thresholding method specific for MPSL images. They observed that, although the lesion intensities distribution $f_l(x)$ is unknown, the distribution $f_s(x)$ of the skin correspond to a Gaussian-like distribution:

$$f_s(x) = Ae^{\frac{-(x-\mu_s)^2}{2\sigma_s^2}}, \tag{5}$$

where, μ_s is the mean value of healthy skin pixel intensities. Being f_{l+s} the distribution of grayscale intensities of the whole image, μ_s is determined by the corresponding intensity value of the highest peak of f_{l+s}. Since $f_{l+s} = f_l + f_s$, and μ_l

(the mean value of lesion pixels) always is lower than μ_s, this distribution can be approximated as:

$$f_{l+s}(x) = \begin{cases} f_s(x), & x \geq \mu_s, \\ f_l(x) + f_s(x), & x < \mu_s. \end{cases} \tag{6}$$

Therefore, based on this assumption, the skin pixels distribution can be estimated as:

$$\widetilde{f}_s(x) = \begin{cases} f_{l+s}(2\mu_s - x), & x < \mu_s, \\ f_{l+s}(x), & x \geq \mu_s, \end{cases} \tag{7}$$

and, consequently, the lesion pixels distribution as:

$$\widetilde{f}_l(x) = f_{l+s}(x) - \widetilde{f}_s(x). \tag{8}$$

Finally, the means $\widetilde{E}(X_s)$ and $\widetilde{E}(X_l)$ of the distributions $\widetilde{f}_s(x)$ and $\widetilde{f}_l(x)$, respectively, are used for the computation of the threshold T as follows:

$$T = \frac{\widetilde{E}(X_s) + \widetilde{E}(X_l)}{2}, \tag{9}$$

and, as in the Otsu's method, the pixels with values lower than the computed threshold, are segmented as lesion pixels.

Figure 2 illustrates the performance of the above mentioned thresholding-based segmentation methods. As can be observed, these low-complexity algorithms are able to determine the lesion area, suffering from boundary definition inaccuracies caused by hair. Also, it is important to observe that the method proposed by Alcon et al. is negatively affected by the lack of a post-processing method to eliminate undesired thresholded areas. Finally, Fig. 2(i) shows the difference between Otsu and Alcon et al. results, obtained by thresholding different regions of the histogram.

3.1.2 Multi-Direction GVF Snake Method

Some researchers have proposed to use Snakes (or Active-Contours) methods to segmented MPSL images, instead of a thresholding method [19]. These methods usually start by smoothing the image, and as an illustration of such methods we refer to the method proposed by Tang [19]. In this method, the MPSL image is initially smoothed by adaptive anisotropic diffusion filtering. Tang modified the traditional anisotropic diffusion to make it more robust to noise, and more details can be found in [19]. Next, a modification of the traditional GVF (Gradient Vector Flow) snake [26] is used to determine the lesion boundary. The original GVF (u, v) can be determined by the minimization of the following energy function:

$$E_{GVF}(u, v) = \frac{1}{2} \int \int g(|\nabla f|)(u_x^2 + u_y^2 + v_x^2 + v_y^2)$$
$$+ (1 - g(|\nabla f|))((u - f_x)^2 + (v - f_y)^2) dx dy, \tag{10}$$

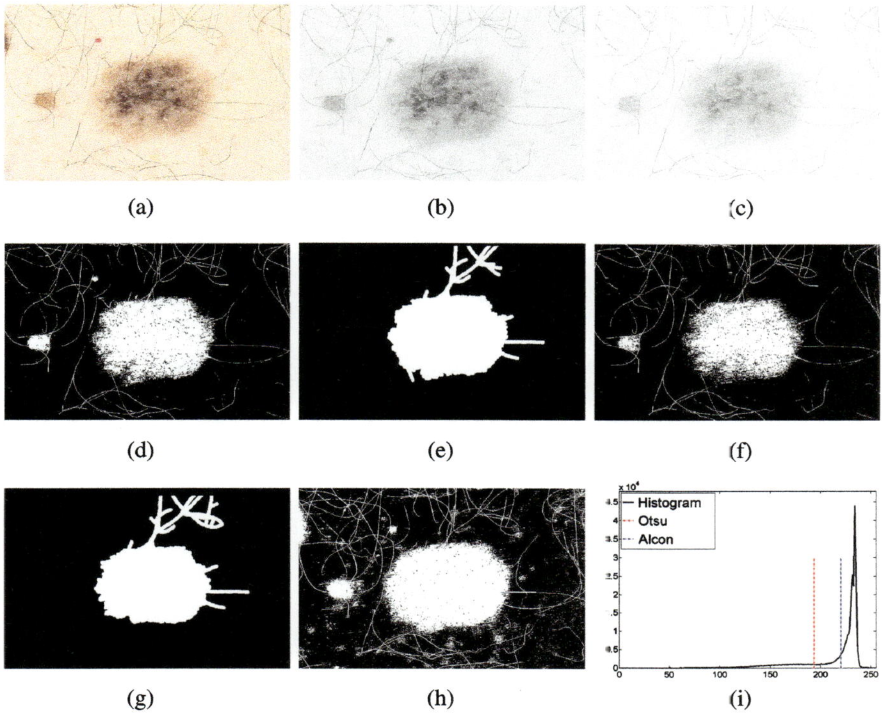

Fig. 2 MPSL image segmentation using thresholding-based methods. (a) The RGB image after pre-processing. (b) Figure (a) after conversion to grayscale. (c) The Red channel of (a). (d) The resultant binary mask of Otsu's method applied to figure (b). (e) The result of applying morphological operation in (d). (f) The resultant binary mask of Otsu's method applied to figure (c). (g) The result of applying morphological operation in (f). (h) The resultant binary mask of Alcon et al. method applied to figure (b). (i) The plot of histogram of figure (b), and the computed Otsu and Alcon thresholds

where, f is an edge map derived from the image, g is an edge-force magnitude:

$$g(|\nabla f|) = \exp\left(-\left(\frac{|\nabla f|}{K}\right)\right), \tag{11}$$

and K is a non-negative smoothing parameter for the field (u, v).

Tang uses a Multi-Directional GVF (MDGVF) in order to create a force-field (u, v) that enforces the snake to converge to the lesion area, and not to spurious image edges. Based on an initialization mask (containing a rough segmentation of the lesion), the author computes the lesion center $(\overline{x}, \overline{y})$ and the direction vector $\mathbf{d}(x, y) = (d_x, d_y)$ at each image pixel (x, y), pointing to the lesion center:

$$d_x = \frac{\overline{x} - x}{\sqrt{(\overline{x} - x)^2 + (\overline{y} - y)^2}}, \tag{12}$$

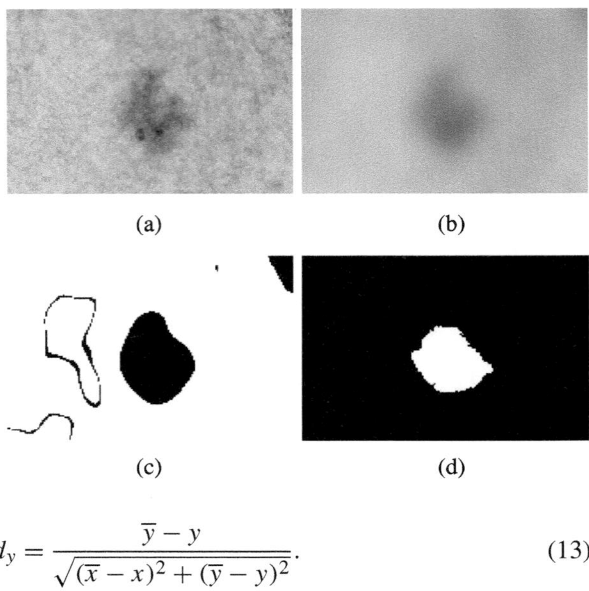

Fig. 3 MPSL image segmentation using multi-direction GVF snake method. (**a**) An example of image after pre-processing and grayscale conversion. (**b**) Image (**a**) after the application of anisotropic diffusion filter. (**c**) The rough segmentation of (**b**). (**d**) The final segmentation after the snake convergence

$$d_y = \frac{\overline{y} - y}{\sqrt{(\overline{x} - x)^2 + (\overline{y} - y)^2}}. \tag{13}$$

After that, the author determines the unitary vector $\mathbf{v}(x, y) = (v_x, v_y)$ for each pixel closer to $\mathbf{d}(x, y)$ by cosine similarity, i.e. $\mathbf{v}(x, y)$ is one of the nine vectors $(-1, -1)$, $(-1, 0)$, $(-1, 1)$, $(0, -1)$, $(0, 0)$, $(0, 1)$, $(1, -1)$, $(1, 0)$ or $(1, 1)$.

Being $I(x, y)$ the grayscale intensity of a pixel (x, y), its respective directional gradient DI can be determined as follows:

$$DI(x, y) = I(x + v_x, y + v_y) - I(x, y). \tag{14}$$

Since often lesions are darker than healthy skin, the negative values of this gradient can be used to determine a new edge-map:

$$F(x, y) = \begin{cases} DI(x, y), & \text{if } DI(x, y) < 0, \\ 0, & \text{otherwise.} \end{cases} \tag{15}$$

Replacing f by F in Eq. (10), a new energy function is obtained to force the snake to converge specifically along the direction of the lesion. To initialize this process, Tang suggests using the Multistage Adaptive Thresholding method [27] to segment the image roughly. In Fig. 3, we present a typical lesion segmentation obtained using this method. The reader may observe that this algorithm handles better artifacts like hair than thresholding-based methods, but unfortunately the lesion boundary is not well determined.

3.2 Multichannel-Based Methods

Although grayscale images have widely being used for segmenting MPSL images, some approaches rely on multichannel images as described in the following sections.

3.2.1 Thresholding-Based Methods

In a similar way that thresholding is used in grayscale MPSL images, we can threshold color images. In this case, thresholds are computed and a binary mask is generated for each channel, and masks are combined to form the final color MPSL image segmentation. However, working with color images adds new concerns. For example, pigmented skin lesions are not easily discriminated from healthy skin on the Green channel (G of the RGB color space), and the color information may disturb instead of benefiting the final results.

So, to facilitate the use of thresholding methods, Cavalcanti and Scharcanski [20] recently proposed a multichannel image representation for MPSL images that maximizes the discrimination between healthy and unhealthy skin regions. The idea is to create a new 3-channel image $\bar{I}_i^N$ based on the normalization of the RGB channels $\bar{I}_i^C$ of the input image, and then use a thresholding algorithm based on Otsu's method to segment it.

The first channel is a representation of the image darkness, relying on the fact that lesion areas are depigmented skin regions. Each pixel is defined as $\bar{I}_1^N(x, y) = 1 - \bar{I}_i^C(x, y)$, i.e. the complement of the normalized Red channel.

The second channel is a texture representation, since local textural variability usually is higher in lesions than in healthy skin areas. Being $\bar{L}$ a normalized Luminance image defined by the average of the three $\bar{I}_i^C$ channels, the textural variability in $\bar{L}(x, y)$ can be quantified by computing $\tau(x, y, \sigma)$ as follows:

$$\tau(x, y, \sigma) = \bar{L}(x, y)\frac{\widetilde{S}(x, y, \sigma)}{S(x, y, \sigma)}, \tag{16}$$

where, $S(x, y, \sigma) = \bar{L}(x, y) * G(\sigma)$ (i.e., the Luminance image $\bar{L}$ is smoothed by a Gaussian filter with standard deviation σ), and $\widetilde{S}(x, y, \sigma)$ represents its complement. In this way, if an image region is dark, its textural information is emphasized; if the region is bright, its textural information is de-emphasized. However, a single Gaussian filter may not be sufficient to capture the textural variability, so $\tau(x, y, \sigma)$ is calculated for different σ values and we select its maximum value at each pixel:

$$T(x, y) = \max_{\sigma}\left[\tau(x, y, \sigma)\right], \quad \sigma \in \{\sigma_1, \sigma_2, \ldots, \sigma_N\}. \tag{17}$$

Finally, the texture variation channel T is normalized, obtaining $\bar{I}_2^N(x, y)$ as follows:

$$\bar{I}_2^N(x, y) = \left(T(x, y) - \min(T)\right)/\left(\max(T) - \min(T)\right). \tag{18}$$

The third channel $\bar{I}_3^N(x, y)$ of the representation describes the local color variation, assuming that healthy and unhealthy skin regions present different color distributions. The Principal Component Analysis (PCA) method is applied on the normalized colors of the image $\bar{I}_i^C(x, y)$, and the first component is retained (i.e. the component that maximizes the local data variance). In this representation, lesion pixels usually have higher variability values than healthy skin pixels, and to detect these lesion pixels in this channel (corresponding to those detected in channels $\bar{I}_1^N$ and $\bar{I}_2^N$), the following PCA property described next is utilized. Since the input data is centered around the mean, and healthy skin pixels often are more frequent in the MPSL image, the projections of the healthy skin pixels on the PCA space tend to generate values nearer to zero than the lesion pixels (i.e., the projected lesion pixels tend to have larger magnitudes, i.e. positive or negative). Therefore, the color variability information C is represented by the pixel projection magnitudes, and the normalization of C generates the $\bar{I}_3^N$ channel:

$$\bar{I}_3^N(x, y) = \big(C(x, y) - \min(C)\big)/\big(\max(C) - \min(C)\big). \tag{19}$$

Also, the $\bar{I}_3^N$ channel is filtered with a 5×5 median filter to reduce the noise. Obtained this multichannel representation, the Otsu's thresholding method (see Sect. 3.1.1) is used to segment the image. Three thresholds th_i are computed, one for each channel $\bar{I}_i^N(x, y)$, and a pixel (x, y) is defined as part of a lesion region (i.e., $\phi(x, y) = 1$) if its value is higher than the threshold th_i in at least two of the three channels:

$$\phi(x, y) = \begin{cases} 1, & \text{if } (\bar{I}_1^N(x, y) > th_1 \wedge \bar{I}_2^N(x, y) > th_2), \\ 1, & \text{if } (\bar{I}_2^N(x, y) > th_2 \wedge \bar{I}_3^N(x, y) > th_3), \\ 1, & \text{if } (\bar{I}_1^N(x, y) > th_1 \wedge \bar{I}_3^N(x, y) > th_3), \\ 0, & \text{otherwise.} \end{cases} \tag{20}$$

As mentioned before (see Sect. 2), after thresholding the remaining skin artifacts (such as freckles and hair) are eliminated more easily. These artifacts usually occur in isolated regions that differ in area and perimeter from skin lesions, since lesions often have larger areas and more irregular boundaries. Therefore, the perimeter and the area of all thresholded connected pixel sets (i.e. where $\phi(x, y) = 1$) are computed, and then this set of regions is partitioned in two clusters. All regions in the cluster with smaller areas (in average) are eliminated, and their correspondent mask pixels are set to $\phi(x, y) = 0$. At the end, the resultant mask is filtered by a 5×5 median filter, eliminating any possible remaining artifacts that may originate rim imperfections.

In Fig. 4, we present the results for all steps of this method, including the multichannel representation generation, the thresholding and post-processing steps. The reader may observe that the lesion boundary is determined with higher precision in comparison to the methods presented previously.

3.2.2 ICA-Based Active-Contours Method

Instead of creating a multichannel representation for a MPSL color image, Cavalcanti et al. [21] recently proposed a segmentation method to be used on the image original color channels. They proposed to use a classical active-contours method (Chan-Vese [28]), followed by morphological operations as a post-processing step.

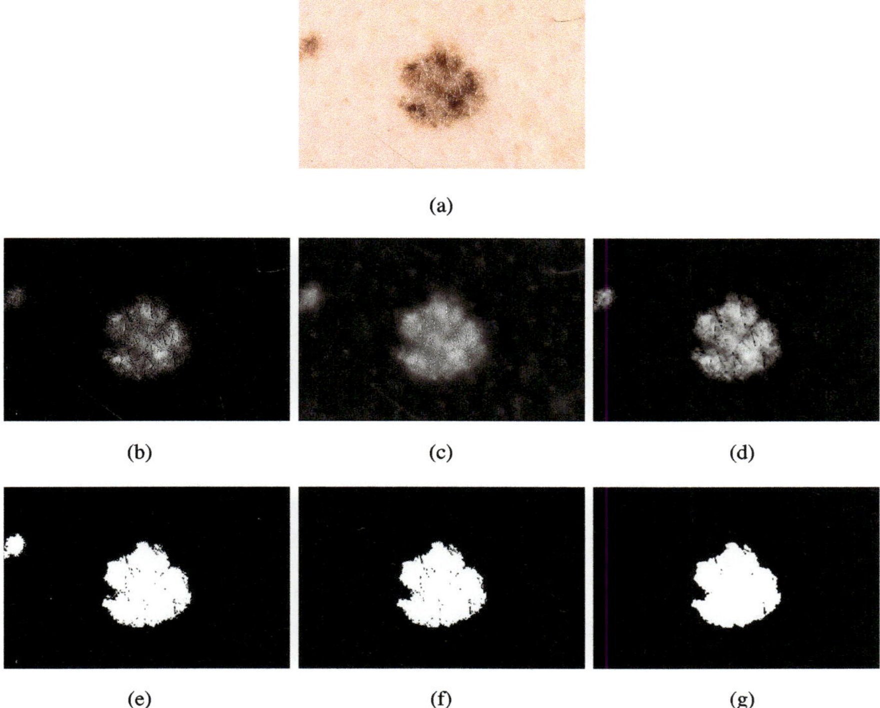

Fig. 4 Segmentation process for the image shown in (a) using thresholding method on a multichannel representation. In (b)–(d), respectively, the $\bar{I}_i^N$ channels representing darkness, texture variation and color variation. In (e)–(g), respectively, binary masks after thresholding, artifacts elimination and filtering

Active-contours methods have already been used to segment pigmented skin lesion images. However, as we seen in Sect. 3.1.2, usually a conversion to a grayscale image precedes the processing stages. Other approaches have been proposed using color images [29], but these algorithms were designed for dermoscopic images, which have different characteristics, and a common drawback of such methods is the difficulty to determine a convenient way to initialize the active-contours algorithm. If the initialization do not indicate the lesion regions with some accuracy, the final segmentation may be incorrect and include healthy skin regions.

Cavalcanti et al. [21] proposed to use independent component analysis (ICA) to generate a reliable binary mask for initializing the active-contours algorithm. They observed that when ICA is applied to a MPSL image, one of the resultant ICA components corresponds mainly to the lesion area, the second component to the healthy skin, and the third component corresponds to noise artifacts. Nevertheless, there is an ordering indeterminacy inherent to the ICA method, and it is not possible to know in advance which component will show the lesion more clearly. However, due to the lesion variability, the histogram of the component that shows more clearly the lesion often has a non-Gaussian histogram (frequently multimodal). The noise artifacts component histogram tends to be non-Gaussian, and the component that shows healthy skin more clearly tends to have a Gaussian histogram. Thus, they estimate the non-Gaussianity of the ICA histogram components with differential entropy, i.e. $\mathcal{J}(X) = |H(X) - H(X_g)|$, where X_g is a Gaussian distributed random variable with the same variance as X. The component that produces the largest differential entropy (i.e., contains the highest non-Gaussianity estimate) is identified as the one containing the lesion information more clearly, and the smallest differential entropy component carries basically healthy skin.

After reordering the channels, the lesion region is best represented in the first channel. Next, the component values are normalized in the range $[0, 1]$, and the Otsu's thresholding method is used (see Sect. 3.1.1) to segment the skin lesion in this channel. Given the ICA results, the lesion information can be emphasized (closer to value 1) or de-emphasized (closer to value 0) in this channel, and consequently the thresholded area may correspond to either, the lesion or the background. To guarantee that the lesion is captured in the thresholded area, the corner pixels (used in the shading attenuation step, that are known to correspond to healthy skin) are tested to check if they are thresholded as '1's or '0's. If most corner pixels are thresholded as '1's, the thresholded area corresponds to healthy skin, and the logical complement is used to obtain the lesion localization mask. In this way, a rough approximation of the lesion area is obtained. Next, the lesion boundary is better approximated and possible artifacts are eliminated with a morphological opening (i.e. the structuring element is a disk with a radius of 3 pixels).

Given this initialization binary mask, Cavalcanti et al. [21] proposed determining the lesion boundary more precisely using the Chan-Vese Active-contours method for vector-valued images [28]. Their method assumes that the color image I_i is formed by two regions of approximately constant intensities c_1 and c_2, separated by a curve C. The lesion localization mask is used as an initialization, indicating approximately the region to be segmented. Afterwards, the active-contours method iteratively tries to minimize the energy function $F(c_1, c_2, C)$ in the color image I_i:

$$F(c_1, c_2, C) = \mu \, length(C) + \lambda_1 \int_{inside(C)} \frac{1}{3} \sum_{i=1}^{3} |I_i(x, y) - c_{1,i}|^2 dxdy$$

$$+ \lambda_2 \int_{outside(C)} \frac{1}{3} \sum_{i=1}^{3} |I_i(x, y) - c_{2,i}|^2 dxdy,$$

where μ, λ_1 and λ_2 are weighting parameters ($\lambda_1 = \lambda_2 = 1$, as suggested in [28], and $\mu = 0.2$). Using the Level-set formulation, it is possible to minimize the energy function embedding the curve C, obtaining the zero level set $C(t) = \{(x, y)|\phi(t, x, y) = 0\}$ of a higher dimensional Level-set function $\phi(t, x, y)$. The evolution of $\phi(t, x, y)$ is given by the following motion Partial Differential Equation:

Fig. 5 Illustration of the segmentation using the ICA-Based Active-Contours method. (**a**) Color image after shading attenuation. (**b**) First re-ordered independent component/channel of image (**a**). (**c**) Lesion localization mask. (**d**) The active-contours segmentation result. (**e**) Final lesion segmentation, after post-processing image (**d**)

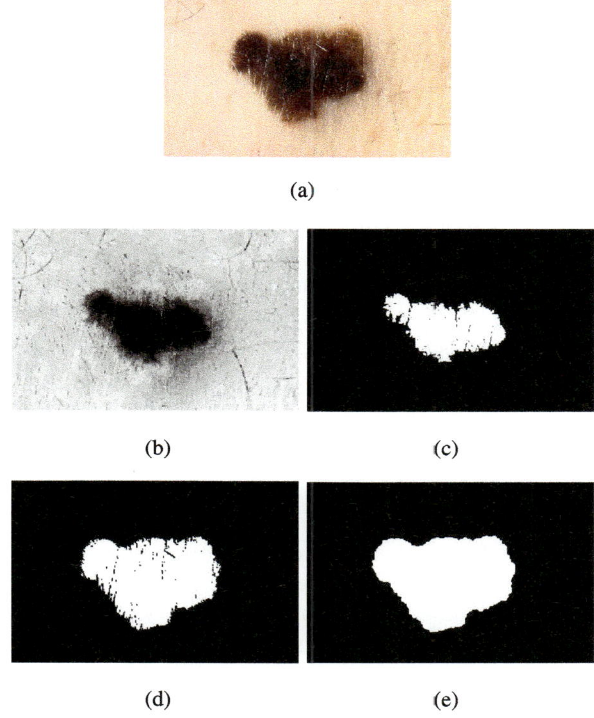

$$\frac{\partial \phi}{\partial t} = \delta_\varepsilon(\phi) \left[\mu \, \mathrm{div}\left(\frac{\nabla \phi}{|\nabla \phi|} \right) - \frac{1}{3} \sum_{i=1}^{3} \lambda_1 \left| I_i(x, y) - c_{1,i} \right|^2 \right.$$

$$\left. + \frac{1}{3} \sum_{i=1}^{3} \lambda_2 \left| I_i(x, y) - c_{2,i} \right|^2 \right], \tag{21}$$

where $\delta_\varepsilon(\phi)$ is the Dirac delta function, $c_{1,i}$ and $c_{2,i}$ are the averages inside and outside of the curve C in the i-th channel I_i, respectively.

It is possible that the final curve C contains regions beyond the lesion area. So, if the number of regions segmented by the Chan-Vese method is higher than one, local artifacts are eliminated. The area and the perimeter of each segmented region are computed, and these values are clustered with K-Means, where $K = 2$. The regions in the cluster with the smaller areas (in average) are eliminated as artifacts and the other regions are kept. The regions kept are hole filled to improve their connectivity, forming the final segmentation mask. The final post-processing step is a morphological dilation (with a disk of 5 pixels of radius as the structuring element).

In Fig. 5, we present the results for all steps of this method. The reader may observe that the initialization mask already do not contain skin artifacts, forcing the active-contours method to a precise determination of the lesion area.

3.3 Comparison of Segmentation Methods Based on Experimental Results

In order to compare the performances of the six state-of-art segmentation methods for MPSL images presented above, we use the same image dataset as in Alcón et al. [17], which contains 152 images that have been collected from the Dermnet dataset [30]. This dataset consists of 107 melanomas and 45 Clark nevi (or atypical nevi), a benign kind of lesion that present similar characteristics to melanomas.

We implemented the shading attenuation step and all the presented algorithms, and processed all the 152 images with these implemented methods. Some examples of segmentation results can be seen in Fig. 6. We also measured the error for each resultant segmentation using the following criterion [6–8]:

$$\varepsilon = \frac{Area(Segmentation \oplus GroundTruth)}{Area(GroundTruth)} \times 100\,\%, \tag{22}$$

where, *Segmentation* is the result of the method in test, *GroundTruth* is the manual segmentation of the same lesion, $Area(S)$ denotes the number of pixels indicated as lesion in the segmentation result S, and $\oplus$ indicates the exclusive-OR, operation that gives the pixels for which the *Segmentation* and *GroundTruth* disagree.

The average error obtained by each segmentation method is presented in Table 1. We also included a synopsis of the six segmentation methods tested in Table 1. As can be seen, the only method that uses color information (ICA-Based Active-Contours Method) generates the smallest error segmentation, in average. Although the methods based on the Otsu's Thresholding Method are not computationally as intense as the method based on active-contours, those methods appear in the sequence, as those with the smallest segmentation errors (multichannel representation appears to be more effective than the methods based on grayscale images). The thresholding method proposed by Alcón et al. and the Multi-Direction GVF Snake method were ranked last, since these methods presented higher segmentation errors. It shall be observed that these methods do not have a post-processing step. Analyzing the segmentation results visually (see Fig. 6), we may observe that the lack of a segmentation post-processing step to eliminate artifacts usually generate segmentations larger than the lesion itself.

Besides the average errors, we present in Table 2 the percentage of images in the database that had lesion segmentation errors lower than 5 %, 10 %, 20 %, 30 % and 40 %, respectively. As can be seen, the Otsu's thresholding method applied on grayscale images tends to be more accurate, but potentially it also can generate larger segmentation errors than the ICA-Based Active-Contours method (the only method that uses color MPSL images). On the other hand, the ICA-Based Active-Contours method tends to be more reliable in the sense that it is less likely to produce large segmentation errors, and obtained experimentally the most accurate lesion segmentation results (in average).

Considering the results presented in Tables 1 and 2, we can infer that color can contribute to improve the segmentation of a MPSL image. Although methods based on one single channel may segment accurately some MPSL images, in average the

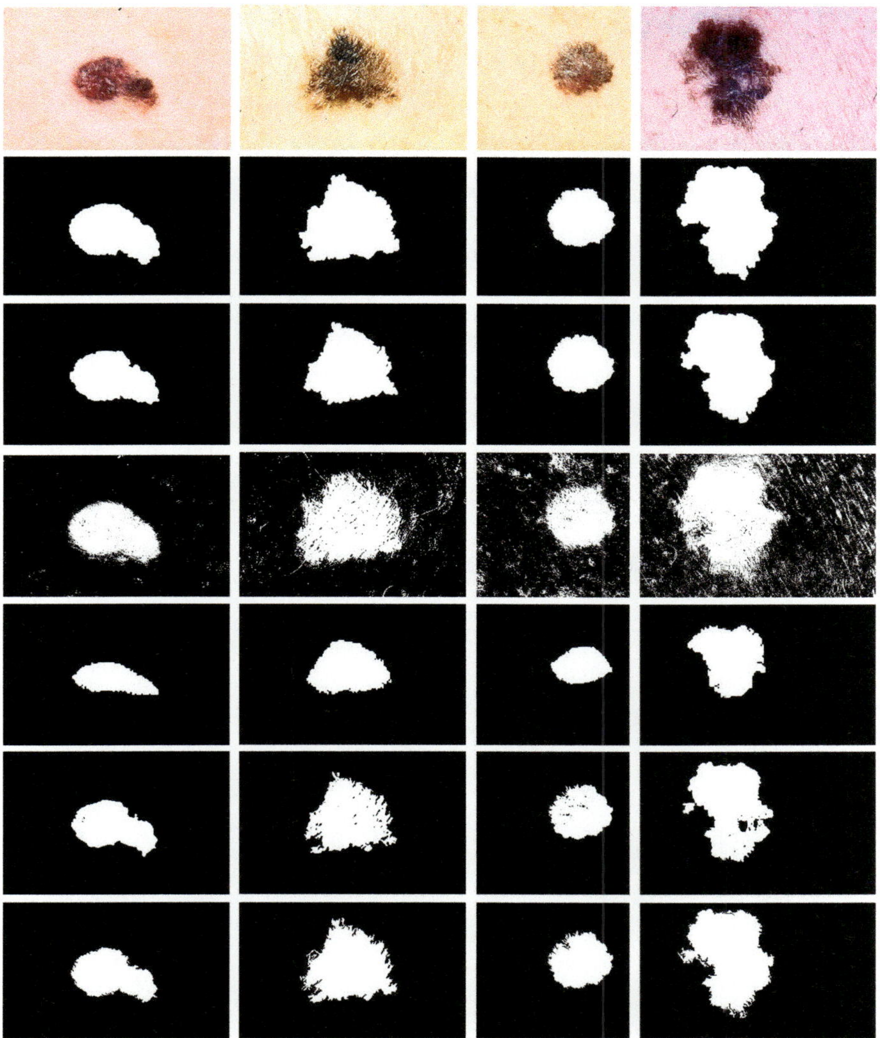

Fig. 6 Examples of MPSL images and their respective segmentation results for the six presented methods. In the *1st. line*, the color images (after shading attenuation). *From 2nd. to 7th. lines*, respectively, results of Otsu's Thresholding Method on Grayscale, Otsu's Thresholding Method on the Red Channel, Alcón et al. Thresholding Method, Multi-Direction GVF Snake Method, Thresholding Method on a Multichannel Representation, and ICA-Based Active-contours Method

color-based method provides more reliable segmentation results. In the next sections, we discuss if the segmentation accuracy is correlated, or not, to the final classification/diagnosis accuracy.

Table 1 Comparison of the six segmentation methods tested for the MPSL image database

Approach	Image type	Post-processing type	Computational cost	ε in average
Otsu's Thresholding Method on Grayscale [15]	Monochromatic	M. Morphology	Low	42.33 %
Otsu's Thresholding Method on the Red Channel [25]	Monochromatic	M. Morphology	Low	38.58 %
Alcón et al. Thresholding Method [17]	Monochromatic	–	Low	165.31 %
Multi-Direction GVF Snake Method [19]	Monochromatic	–	High	59.60 %
Thresholding Method on a Multichannel Representation [20]	Multichannel	M. Morphology	Medium	34.83 %
ICA-Based Active-Contours Method [21]	Multichannel (Color)	M. Morphology	High	28.34 %

Table 2 Segmentation errors in terms of error percentages

Approach	$\varepsilon < 5\,\%$	$\varepsilon < 10\,\%$	$\varepsilon < 20\,\%$	$\varepsilon < 30\,\%$	$\varepsilon < 40\,\%$
ICA-Based Active-Contours Method [21]	3.29 %	29.61 %	73.68 %	86.84 %	94.08 %
Otsu's Thresholding Method on Grayscale [15]	3.29 %	34.87 %	75.66 %	87.50 %	93.42 %
Otsu's Thresholding Method on the Red Channel [25]	1.97 %	27.63 %	67.11 %	83.55 %	93.42 %
Thresholding Method on a Multichannel Representation [20]	1.32 %	4.61 %	43.42 %	69.74 %	81.58 %
Alcón et al. Thresholding Method [17]	0.00 %	0.00 %	8.55 %	16.45 %	25.00 %
Multi-Direction GVF Snake Method [19]	0.00 %	0.00 %	0.00 %	5.92 %	23.03 %

4 Feature Extraction for Skin Lesion Discrimination

Given a MPSL image segmentation, we are able to obtain a classification (or diagnosis) of the acquired pigmented skin lesion. Before obtaining this classification, features representative of the skin lesion must be extracted. Computer-aided diagnosis systems often try to reproduce computationally the ABCD rule [31], which is an acronym referring to the four criteria used in clinical diagnosis, namely: **A**symmetry, **B**order Irregularity, **C**olor Variation and **D**ifferential Structures. Several approaches have been proposed for describing quantitatively the first three criteria [3, 5, 8, 17, 32]. These feature extraction techniques can be used jointly to represent benign and malignant cases better, and discriminate them more effectively. The fourth criterion (i.e. Differential structures) only is visible in dermoscopy images, but to describe quantitatively this lesion characteristic automatically still is challenging.

Since our ultimate goal is to evaluate the influence of image segmentation on the final classification/diagnosis, we will adopt the feature extraction and classification scheme proposed specifically for MPSL images by Cavalcanti and Scharcanski [20]. In the following sections we present the 52 features that have been used in their ABCD rule implementation, also including features that were proposed by other authors. In terms of terminology, it is important to clarify that images $\bar{I}_i^C$ and $\bar{I}_i^N$ refer to a normalized color image and to the multichannel image representation presented in Sect. 3.2.1, respectively.

4.1 Features Used for Lesion Asymmetry Characterization

The goal of these features is to quantify the lesion shape, in special the asymmetry of the lesion in relation to the principal axes. The major axis L_1 of the lesion is aligned with its longest diameter, passing through its center; the minor axis L_2 is orthogonal to L_1 and also passes through the shape center. The features utilized are the following:

f_1: Solidity: the ratio between the lesion area (A) and its convex hull area [17];

f_2: Extent: the ratio between the lesion area and its bounding box area [17];

f_3: Equivalent diameter: $4A/(L_1\pi)$ [5, 17];

f_4: Circularity: $4\pi A/(L_1 p)$, where p is the lesion perimeter [17];

f_5: The ratio between the principal axes (L_2/L_1) [5, 17];

f_6: The ratio between sides of the lesion bounding box [17];

f_7: The ratio between the lesion perimeter p and its area A [3];

f_8: $(B_1 - B_2)/A$, where, B_1 and B_2 are the areas in each side of axis L_1;

f_9: Similar to f_8, but makes use of the shorter axis L_2;

f_{10}: $B1/B2$ with respect to the axis L_1;

f_{11}: Similar to f_{10}, but makes use of the shorter axis L_2.

4.2 Features Used for Lesion Boundary Irregularity Characterization

The boundary sharpness is quantified by the magnitude of the gradient $|\vec{\nabla} \bar{I}_i^N|$ at each pixel using the Sobel operator [20]. However, instead of using pixels only at the lesion rim, we analyze pixels in an extended (dilated) rim[1] [17]. Consequently,

---

[1]The rim is dilated by 2 pixels, producing a 5 pixels wide region centered at the lesion rim, as suggested in [17].

lesions that have a smooth boundary (usually nevi) are better characterized. Also, the lesion boundary dilation makes the boundary representation more robust to the inaccuracies of the segmentation process. To characterize the lesion boundary irregularity, the following features are used [20]:

$f_{12}-f_{14}$: Average gradient magnitude of the pixels in the lesion extended rim [17], in each one of the three $\bar{I}_i^N$ channels;
$f_{15}-f_{17}$: Variance of the gradient magnitude of the pixels in the lesion extended rim [17], in each one of the three $\bar{I}_i^N$ channels;

The lesion rim irregularity is characterized in the ABCD rule by dividing the rim in 8 symmetric regions [31]. In addition to the two principal axes L_1 and L_2, two additional axes are obtained by rotating by 45 degrees these orthogonal axes. Therefore, 8 symmetric regions $R = 1, \ldots, 8$ are generated. For each channel $\bar{I}_i^N$, the average gradient magnitudes of the extended rim pixels $\mu_{R,i}$ ($R = 1, \ldots, 8$) are computed. Therefore, 6 more features are calculated:

$f_{18}-f_{20}$: Average of the 8 $\mu_{R,i}$ values in each one of the three $\bar{I}_i^N$ channels;
$f_{21}-f_{23}$: Variance of the 8 $\mu_{R,i}$ values in each one of the three $\bar{I}_i^N$ channels;

4.3 Features Used for Lesion Color Variation Characterization

These features quantify the color variation in the lesion, and the following measurements can be utilized for this purpose [20]:

$f_{24}-f_{27}$: Maximum, minimum, mean and variance of the pixels intensities inside the lesion segment in the color variation channel $\bar{I}_3^N$;
$f_{28}-f_{39}$: Maximum, minimum, mean and variance of the pixels intensities inside the lesion segment in each one of three original $\bar{I}_i^C$ channels;
$f_{40}-f_{42}$: Ratios between mean values of the tree original $\bar{I}_i^C$ channels: $mean(\bar{I}_1^C)/mean(\bar{I}_2^C)$, $mean(\bar{I}_1^C)/mean(\bar{I}_3^C)$ and $mean(\bar{I}_2^C)/mean(\bar{I}_3^C)$, considering only pixels inside the lesion segment.

Physicians usually identify six distinct hues in skin lesions: white, red, light and dark brown, blue-gray, and black [31]. Lesions containing more of these hues are more likely to be malignant. The lesion color variability can be quantified by computing the occurrence of these typical hues within a lesion segment. Given a pixel in the lesion segment, the nearest reference color (associated with a typical hue, see Table 3 [17]) is found by the Euclidean distance to the pixel color in $\bar{I}_i^C$. A hue occurrence counter is created, one cell per typical hue. For each lesion pixel, the nearest typical hue counter is increased by 1. Finally, typical hues counters are normalized/divided by the lesion area A, and generate the 6 additional features $f_{43}-f_{48}$.

Table 3 Six possible colors of a lesion on the RGB color space

Color	Red	Green	Blue
White	1	1	1
Red	0.8	0.2	0.2
Light Brown	0.6	0.4	0
Dark Brown	0.2	0	0
Blue-Gray	0.2	0.6	0.6
Black	0	0	0

4.4 Features Used for Lesion Differential Structures Characterization

The lesion differential structures refer to submacroscopic morphologic and vascular structures only visible in dermoscope images. In an attempt to extract the characteristics of these structures also on a macroscopic image, differences between benign and malignant lesions can be measured using texture features. Cavalcanti and Scharcanski [20] propose to extract the 4 features $f_{49}-f_{52}$, namely the maximum, minimum, mean and variance of the pixels intensities inside the lesion segment to represent the textural variation in the channel $\bar{I}_2^N$.

4.5 Feature Extraction Summary

Even for specialized physicians the discrimination of benign from malignant pigmented skin lesions may not be an easy task, and the development of techniques that facilitate this job is a current research topic. In the previous sections, we presented 52 features that help in this task, but readers can probably find additional (or even alternative) features in literature, and probably new features will be proposed in the coming years as this research area develops. The ultimate goal is to represent image lesion characteristics to could facilitate the early classification/diagnosis and reduce the number of deaths caused by these lesions.

Another important issue when dealing with the selection of feature sets is the adoption of automatic (or interactive) feature selection algorithms. Some authors of classification approaches for pigmented skins lesions [5, 15, 17] suggest using a method to select the best features as those that help most the MPSL image class discrimination. However, this feature selection procedure can be tricky. Pigmented skin lesions have a large variability in terms of characteristics, and the discrimination between a malignant and a benign case can be determined by only 1 or 2 features. If these features have been eliminated because they did not seem to be important on a given training set, malignant cases can be incorrectly classified as benign, leading to costly false negatives.

5 Classification of Pigmented Skin Lesion Images

After extracting the features that characterize each MPSL image, we can use these data to obtain a final classification (or diagnosis) of the imaged lesion. We discuss how this information is processed in the following sections.

5.1 Feature Normalization

The extracted features may have values in different ranges. Some of the proposed approaches do not perform feature normalization [8, 17]. However, classifiers tend to be more efficient if these feature values are normalized and represented in the same range (i.e., the feature values are scaled to fall in a specified range), therefore we adopt this normalization step in our work.

This feature value scaling is performed based on the mean and standard deviation of the captured feature values [5, 20, 32]. Among the possible feature normalization options [32, 33], we chose to normalize the feature values using the well known z-score transformation [33]:

$$Z_{i,j} = \frac{((v_{i,j} - \mu_j)/(3\sigma_j) + 1)}{2}, \tag{23}$$

where, $v_{i,j}$ is the value of the jth feature of the ith sample (image), μ_j and σ_j are the mean and standard deviation of the jth feature, respectively. After the z-score transformation, most of the $Z_{i,j}$ values are in the [0, 1] range. The out-of-range values are saturated to either 0 or 1.

5.2 Defining Training Sets

Classification techniques are commonly used in machine learning. The validation test requires the definition of training sets, and two methodologies are usually applied, namely: cross-validation and holdout validation [34]. The cross-validation method divides the samples in S portions, and $S - 1$ portions are used for training while the remaining portion is used for testing. This process is repeated until all the samples have been evaluated. In the holdout validation, part of the samples in each class (benign or malignant) are randomly selected and used for training, and the remaining samples are used for testing. Often, up to half of the initial sample set is used for testing. The holdout validation method was used in our experiments described in Sect. 6.

However, a common limitation of the public domain MPSL datasets is the relatively small number of cases, specially in the benign class (which often leads to unbalanced training sets). So, in addition to the selection of representative samples, we often need to balance and extend the training sets. One popular alternative is to add new training samples using the Smoothed Bootstrap Resampling method [20, 35]. This method is used when there are not enough samples to guarantee the statistical significance of the data set. In this case, the original samples are randomly selected, and new ones are created by adding a small amount of zero-centered noise to their feature values, enlarging the data set [35]. In our experiments (see Sect. 6), we used zero mean Gaussian noise, with $\sigma = 0.1$, and made sure to obtain at least 2500 samples for each class (5000 samples in total) for a two class problem.

5.3 Classification Methods

After the feature normalization and the training samples selection steps, the generated data is the input used to train a classification method. For the classification of pigmented skin lesions images (macroscopic or dermoscopic), Support Vector Machines (SVM) is frequently utilized [5, 16]. However, due to the complex class shapes generated by the feature data, determining an adequate kernel and its parameters often is a difficult task. Artificial Neural Networks [15, 36] suffer from a similar limitation, determining the number of layers in multilayer perceptrons and their characteristics is critical, and may increase or decrease the final accuracy significantly. However, techniques such Decision and Regression Trees [17] usually are less computationally intensive, and the parameters can be determined automatically. However, despite of their relatively simplicity, such classifier used alone hardly obtain the desirable accuracy levels by state-of-the-art of MPSL classification schemes.

In our experiments, where we try to relate segmentation and classification performance, we used a Nearest Neighbor Classifier (KNN) with $K = 1$. This algorithm is very simple, where each sample/image is assigned to its neighbor class using the Euclidean Distance in feature space. This method was chosen for its simplicity and because it has been already used successfully in pigmented skin lesion image classification research [20, 36, 37].

6 Discussion of Experimental Evidences: Pigmented Skin Lesion Segmentation and Its Influence on the Lesion Classification and Diagnosis

In the previous sections, we discuss the procedures utilized to obtain a classification/diagnosis for a MPSL image, from the pre-processing steps to the final classification. Now, we wish to evaluate the influence of the segmentation methods in the final lesion classification/diagnosis.

Recall that the Alcón et al. dataset used in our experiments (see Sect. 3.3) contains 107 melanoma images (malignant cases) and 45 Clark nevi images (benign cases). In Tables 4, 5, 6 and 7 we present the classification results for these 152

Table 4 Comparison of classification results in average

Approach	Sensitivity	Specificity	Accuracy
Alcón et al. Thresholding Method [17]	92.56 %	89.16 %	91.55 %
Otsu's Thresholding Method on Grayscale [15]	93.89 %	83.91 %	90.93 %
ICA-Based Active-Contours Method [21]	92.95 %	85.60 %	90.78 %
Thresholding Method on a Multichannel Representation [20]	93.91 %	83.29 %	90.76 %
Multi-Direction GVF Snake Method [19]	92.34 %	86.89 %	90.72 %
Otsu's Thresholding Method on the Red Channel [25]	94.17 %	80.36 %	90.08 %

Table 5 Best classification results in terms of sensitivity

Approach	Sensitivity	Specificity	Accuracy
Otsu's Thresholding Method on the Red Channel [25]	99.07 %	75.56 %	92.11 %
Alcón et al. Thresholding Method [17]	99.07 %	75.56 %	92.11 %
Multi-Direction GVF Snake Method [19]	98.13 %	86.67 %	94.74 %
Thresholding Method on a Multichannel Representation [20]	98.13 %	86.67 %	94.74 %
ICA-Based Active-Contours Method [21]	98.13 %	84.44 %	94.08 %
Otsu's Thresholding Method on Grayscale [15]	97.20 %	80.00 %	92.11 %

Table 6 Best classification results in terms of specificity

Approach	Sensitivity	Specificity	Accuracy
Alcón et al. Thresholding Method [17]	92.52 %	97.78 %	94.08 %
ICA-Based Active-Contours Method [21]	92.52 %	95.56 %	93.42 %
Multi-Direction GVF Snake Method [19]	87.85 %	93.33 %	89.47 %
Thresholding Method on a Multichannel Representation [20]	93.46 %	91.11 %	92.76 %
Otsu's Thresholding Method on Grayscale [15]	94.39 %	88.89 %	92.76 %
Otsu's Thresholding Method on the Red Channel [25]	94.39 %	88.89 %	92.76 %

images obtained by different state-of-the-art methods. In each one of these Tables, we present the Sensitivity (i.e, the percentage of MPSL images correctly classified in the malignant class), Specificity (i.e., the percentage of MPSL images correctly classified in the benign class) and Accuracy (i.e., the percentage of MPSL images correctly classified overall, considering all images).

Since the training sample selection process is random (see Sect. 5.2), and may not assure that the selected samples represent well the characteristics of both classes, we considered as representative all the 50 training sets obtained in 50 random trails, as well as the 50 classification results corresponding to each one of these training sets.

Table 7 Best classification results in terms of accuracy

Approach	Sensitivity	Specificity	Accuracy
Alcón et al. Thresholding Method [17]	98.13 %	88.89 %	95.39 %
Thresholding Method on a Multichannel Representation [20]	98.13 %	86.67 %	94.74 %
ICA-Based Active-Contours Method [21]	97.20 %	88.89 %	94.74 %
Multi-Direction GVF Snake Method [19]	97.20 %	88.89 %	94.74 %
Otsu's Thresholding Method on Grayscale [15]	96.26 %	88.89 %	94.08 %
Otsu's Thresholding Method on the Red Channel [25]	94.39 %	88.89 %	92.76 %

That is, we computed 50 times: (a) the training samples selection, (b) the Smoothed Bootstrap Resampling method, and (c) the Nearest Neighbor classifier results, so that our experimental results are statistically relevant. The final classification performance is measured based on these 50 trials.

We present the Accuracy, Specificity and Sensitivity averages of the 50 obtained results in Table 4. In Tables 5, 6 and 7, we present the best classification results for each segmentation method tested (in terms of Sensitivity, Specificity and Accuracy, respectively). As can be seen, these segmentation methods were ranked based on their segmentation (see Sect. 3) and classification errors, but their segmentation and classification rankings differ. This indicates that the MPSL image feature set describes the lesions well, representing well their morphology even if the segmentation is not as precise as would be desirable. Additionally, these experimental results show that better feature extraction techniques that could take advantage of more accurate segmentations are needed, achieving classification results that are more accurate.

It shall be observed that our classification results indicate accuracies higher than 90 % (in average), independent of the selected segmentation algorithm. These accuracies are higher than the diagnosis accuracies obtained by trained physicians in telemedicine, which range between 31 % to 85 % according to the literature [13].

7 Summary and Future Trends

In this chapter, we reviewed the procedures used for classifying or diagnosing a pigmented skin lesion from a macroscopic image. Given the acquired color image, we showed how to eliminate shading effects, determine the lesion boundaries and some of the important lesion characteristics, and how to obtain the correct lesion classification as a (malignant) melanoma or a (benign) nevus.

The importance of using color also is outlined in this work, since the use of color can enhance the MPSL image segmentation precision. It shall be observed that the classification accuracies obtained in such segmentation and classification schemes already can be higher than the diagnosis accuracies obtained by trained physicians in telemedicine. Although the segmentation results do not correlate well with the final classification accuracies, we believe that in future new features can be developed to make better use of more precise segmentations, leading even higher classification accuracies.

In particular, we believe that such automatic MPSL image analysis schemes will contribute to increase the reliability of telemedicine. Consequently, the access to MPSL image prescreening systems shall be increase in the near future, which will contribute to improve the current early skin cancer detection rates, the skin cancer patient prognosis, and also it shall help increase the efficiency of the medical care systems.

References

1. World Health Organization. How commom is skin cancer? http://www.who.int/uv/faq/skincancer/en/index1.html
2. Rao BK, Marghoob AA, Stolz W, Kopf AW, Slade J, Wasti Q, Schoenbach SP, De-David M, Bart RS (1997) Can early malignant melanoma be differentiated from atypical melanocytic nevi by in vivo techniques? Skin Res Technol 3(1):8–14
3. Fikrle T, Pizinger K (2007) Digital computer analysis of dermatoscopical images of 260 melanocytic skin lesions; perimeter/area ratio for the differentiation between malignant melanomas and melanocytic nevi. J Eur Acad Dermatol Venereol 21:48–55
4. Mayer J (1997) Systematic review of the diagnostic accuracy of dermatoscopy in detecting malignant melanoma. Med J Aust 167:206–210
5. Celebi ME, Kingravi HA, Uddin B, Iyatomi H, Aslandogan YA, Stoecker WV, Moss RH (2007) A methodological approach to the classification of dermoscopy images. Comput Med Imaging Graph 31(6):362–373
6. Celebi ME, Kingravi HA, Iyatomi H, Aslandogan YA, Stoecker WV, Moss RH, Malters JM, Grichnik JM, Marghoob AA, Rabinovitz HS, Menzies SW (2008) Border detection in dermoscopy images using statistical region merging. Skin Res Technol 14:347–353
7. Gomez DD, Butakoff C, Ersboll BK, Stoecker W (2008) Independent histogram pursuit for segmentation of skin lesions. IEEE Trans Biomed Eng 55:157–161
8. Iyatomi H, Oka H, Celebi M, Hashimoto M, Hagiwara M, Tanaka M, Ogawa K (2008) An improved internet-based melanoma screening system with dermatologist-like tumor area extraction algorithm. Comput Med Imaging Graph 32(7):566–579
9. Zhou H, Schaefer G, Sadka A, Celebi M (2009) Anisotropic mean shift based fuzzy c-means segmentation of dermoscopy images. IEEE J Sel Top Signal Process 3:26–34
10. Zhou H, Schaefer G, Celebi ME, Lin F, Liu T (2011) Gradient vector flow with mean shift for skin lesion segmentation. Comput Med Imaging Graph 35(2):121–127
11. Skvara H, Teban L, Fiebiger M, Binder M, Kittler H (2005) Limitations of dermoscopy in the recognition of melanoma. Arch Dermatol 141:155–160
12. Massone C, Wurm EMT, Hofmann-Wellenhof R, Soyer HP (2008) Teledermatology: an update. Semin Cutan Med Surg 27:101–105
13. Whited JD (2006) Teledermatology research review. Int J Dermatol 45:220–229
14. Manousaki AG, Manios AG, Tsompanaki EI, Panayiotides JG, Tsiftsis DD, Kostaki AK, Tosca AD (2006) A simple digital image processing system to aid in melanoma diagnosis in an everyday melanocytic skin lesion unit: a preliminary report. Int J Dermatol 45:402–410
15. Ruiz D, Berenguer VJ, Soriano A, Martin J (2008) A cooperative approach for the diagnosis of the melanoma. In: Proceedings of the 30th annual international conference of the IEEE engineering in medicine and biology society (EMBC), vol 2008, pp 5144–5147

16. Tabatabaie K, Esteki A, Toossi P (2009) Extraction of skin lesion texture features based on independent component analysis. Skin Res Technol 15:433–439
17. Alcon JF, Ciuhu C, ten Kate W, Heinrich A, Uzunbajakava N, Krekels G. Siem D, de Haan G (2009) Automatic imaging system with decision support for inspection of pigmented skin lesions and melanoma diagnosis. IEEE J Sel Top Signal Process 3:14–25
18. Parolin A, Herzer E, Jung C (2010) Semi-automated diagnosis of melanoma through the analysis of dermatological images. In: 23rd conference on graphics, patterns and images (SIBGRAPI), pp 71–78
19. Tang J (2009) A multi-direction gvf snake for the segmentation of skin cancer images. Pattern Recognit 42:1172–1179
20. Cavalcanti PG, Scharcanski J (2011) Automated prescreening of pigmented skin lesions using standard cameras. Comput Med Imaging Graph 35(6):481–491
21. Cavalcanti PG, Scharcanski J, Persia LED, Milone DH (2011) An ica-based method for the segmentation of pigmented skin lesions in macroscopic images. In: Proceedings of the 33rd annual international conference of the IEEE engineering in medicine and biology society (EMBC)
22. Tan X, Triggs B (2010) Enhanced local texture feature sets for face recognition under difficult lighting conditions. IEEE Trans Image Process 19:1635–1650
23. Zhou H, Miller P, Zhang J (2011) Age classification using radon transform and entropy based scaling svm. In: Proceedings of the British machine vision conference. BMVA Press, Guildford, pp 28.1–28.12. doi:10.5244/C.25.28
24. Otsu N (1979) A threshold selection method from gray-level histograms. IEEE Trans Syst Man Cybern 9:62–66
25. Cavalcanti P, Yari Y, Scharcanski J (2010) Pigmented skin lesion segmentation on macroscopic images. In: Proceedings of the 25th international conference on image and vision computing, New Zealand
26. Xu C, Prince JL (1998) Snakes, shapes, and gradient vector flow. IEEE Trans Image Process 7(3):359–369
27. Yan F, Zhang H, Kube CR (2005) A multistage adaptive thresholding method. Pattern Recognit Lett 26:1183–1191
28. Chan TF, Sandberg BY, Vese LA (2000) Active contours without edges for vector-valued images. J Vis Commun Image Represent 11(2):130–141
29. Silveira M, Nascimento J, Marques J, Marcal A, Mendonca T, Yamauchi S, Maeda J, Rozeira J (2009) Comparison of segmentation methods for melanoma diagnosis in dermoscopy images. IEEE J Sel Top Signal Process 3:35–45
30. Dermnet skin disease image atlas. http://www.dermnet.com
31. Nachbar F, Stolz W, Merkle T, Cognetta AB, Vogt T, Landthaler M, Bilek P, Braun-Falco O, Plewig G (1994) The abcd rule of dermatoscopy: high prospective value in the diagnosis of doubtful melanocytic skin lesions. J Am Acad Dermatol 30(4):551–559
32. Ganster H, Pinz P, Rohrer R, Wildling E, Binder M, Kittler H (2001) Automated melanoma recognition. IEEE Trans Med Imaging 20:233–239
33. Aksoy S, Haralick RM (2000) Probabilistic vs. geometric similarity measures for image retrieval. In: Proceedings of the IEEE conference on computer vision and pattern recognition, 13–15 June 2002, vol 2, pp 357–362
34. Bishop CM (2007) Pattern recognition and machine learning, 1st edn. Information science and statistics. Springer, Berlin
35. Young GA (1990) Alternative smoothed bootstraps. J R Stat Soc, Ser B, Methodol 52(3):477–484
36. Dreiseitl S, Ohno-Machado L, Kittler H, Vinterbo S, Billhardt H, Binder M (2001) A comparison of machine learning methods for the diagnosis of pigmented skin lesions. J Biomed Inform 34:28–36
37. Burroni M, Corona R, Dell'Eva G, Sera F, Bono R, Puddu P, Perotti R, Nobile F, Andreassi L, Rubegni P (2004) Melanoma computer-aided diagnosis: reliability and feasibility study. Clin Cancer Res 10:1881–1886

Color and Spatial Features Integrated Normalized Distance for Density Based Border Detection in Dermoscopy Images

Sinan Kockara, Mutlu Mete, and Sait Suer

Abstract Dermoscopy is the major imaging modality used in the diagnosis of melanoma and other pigmented skin lesions. Automated assessment tools for dermoscopy images have become an important research field mainly because of inter- and intra-observer inconsistencies at interpretation of the same image. Automated detection of lesion borders is very important step in dermoscopy image analysis. One of the highest accuracy rates in the automated lesion border detection field is achieved by Fast Density Based Lesion Detection (FDBLD), which is based on density based clustering of pixel-of-interest. In addition to low border detection error, FDBLD removes redundant computations in well-known spatial density based clustering algorithm DBSCAN; thus, in turn it accelerates clustering process considerably. However, FDBLD is designed to run only on binary images; thus, it requires pre-processing step to convert color image in to a binary image. Furthermore, very important color information in dermoscopy images falls into disuse.

In this study, we develop a modified FDBLD by introducing a new distance measure called Normalized Distance. Our method (ND- FDBLD) improves the efficiency of lesion detection by plugging Normalized Distance into FDBLD. This in turn removes dependency of FDBLD to preprocessing step and improves its accuracy. Moreover, developed distance measure helped involve both color and position dependencies in FDBLD. Both FDBLD and ND-FDBLD methods, in experiments, are tested on the same set of dermoscopy images. ND-FDBLD method is compared not only against FDBLD but also against dermatologists' drawn ground truth lesion border images. Results revealed that new algorithm is more accurate and efficient than FDBLD on 75 % of 100 dermoscopy images. On 23 % of images both our method and FDBLD performed the same accuracy rates. FDBLD had better accuracy than ND-FDBLD only on two images. In parallel to these results, ND-FDBLD

S. Kockara (✉) · S. Suer
Department of Computer Science, University of Central Arkansas, 201 Donaghey Ave., Conway, AR 72035, USA
e-mail: skockara@uca.edu

M. Mete
Department of Computer Science and Information Systems, Texas A&M University—Commerce, Commerce, TX 75429, USA

M.E. Celebi, G. Schaefer (eds.), *Color Medical Image Analysis*, 41
Lecture Notes in Computational Vision and Biomechanics 6,
DOI 10.1007/978-94-007-5389-1_3, © Springer Science+Business Media Dordrecht 2013

generates more accurate results than FDBLD compared to dermatologists' drawn ground truth images.

1 Introduction

Skin cancer is one of the most common cancer types. Three most widely seen skin cancer types are melanoma, basal cell cancer, and squamous cell cancer which are named after the type of skin cells from which cancer arises [1]. Skin cancer is the most commonly diagnosed cancer type and it is rarely fatal, except for melanoma [2]. Melanoma is the most rapidly increasing cancer in the world and is the sixth most common cancer in the US [3]. In 2010, there were estimated 68,130 new cases in the US. Unfortunately, 8,700 of these cases were fatal [1]. Although survival rate is increasing, death rate from malignant melanoma is exponentially increasing too [3]. Early diagnosis is crucial for the treatment, because malignant melanoma is very invasive when it affects melanocyte. Melanoma develops in the epidermis. An often-used mnemonic for early signs of melanoma is "ABCDE rule", where A corresponds to asymmetry, B is borders (irregular), C is color, D corresponds to diameter, and E indicates characteristics of evolving over time. Since it is found between the outer layer of the skin (the epidermis) and the next layer (the dermis), it is clearly visible by human eyes. The diseased area can be cured by a surgical excision operation.

2 Dermoscopy Image Analysis

Dermoscopy is one of the major imaging techniques for detecting skin lesion area. It is found that, by using dermoscopy techniques, the sensitivity of finding the lesion area increases up to 20 % [4]. Dermoscopy images give dermatologists confidence in determining the lesion. Combining dermoscopy and computer aided diagnosis (CAD) techniques is a very important and active research field. In order to prevent time loss and intra- and inter-observer variations, researchers try to utilize computerized techniques. The borders of most melanomas are often indistinct which makes visual identification very difficult. Over time, the lesion may grow or the pigmentation in the lesion may darken. To evaluate changes in the lesion by time, the previous border of the same lesion must be compared side by side with the current border of the same lesion. Therefore, delineating lesion borders on dermoscopy images are critical. In the current practice, dermatologists visually check the dermoscopy images and manually or virtually draw the lesion border which is a tedious and error-prone process. Moreover, the delineated lesion border drawn by various dermatologists may not be the same. Sometimes this difference may reach up to 24 % [5]. Motivated by these facts, CAD techniques are developed to help dermatologists to reduce possible differences, and standardize the results by alleviating inter- and intra-observer variations, and accelerate the process [5, 6].

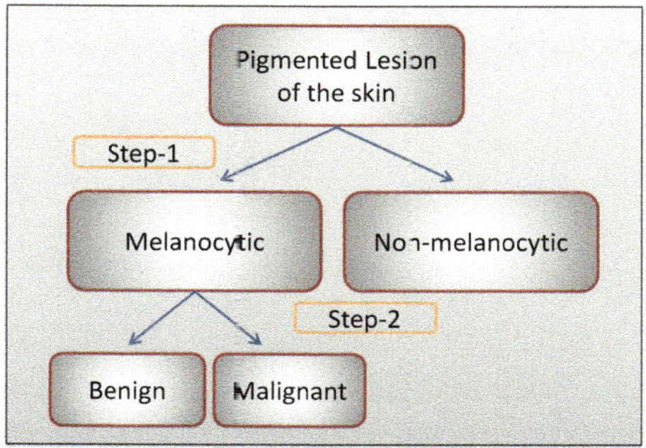

Fig. 1 Two-step procedure for classifying the lesion area in dermoscopy [12]

At the first stage of dermoscopy image analysis, border detection is usually applied [7, 8] to detect other features more accurately. Since human eye does not perceive minor color and shape changes, help of CAD techniques is beneficial at this step. There are many factors that make automated border detection complex. For instance, low contrast between the surrounding skin and the lesion, fuzzy and irregular lesion border, and intrinsic artifacts such as cutaneous features (air bubbles, blood vessels, hairs and black frames) can be named [5]. According to Celebi et al. [5] automated border detection can be divided into four sections: pre-processing, segmentation, post-processing, and evaluation. The pre-processing step involves color space transformations [7], contrast enhancement [9] and artifacts removal [10]. The segmentation step involves partitioning of an image into disjoint regions [11]. The post-processing is used to obtain the lesion border [6]. The evaluation involves the assessment of the border detection results by a dermatologist.

2.1 The ABCDE Rule

Diagnostic steps in dermoscopy are summarized in Fig. 1. After the images are taken by a dermatoscope, the first step is to decide whether or not the lesion is melanocytic. Melanocytes are melanin-producing cells located under the skin's epidermis layer. Once the lesion is identified as melanocytic, the process continues with determining whether it is malignant or benign by using one of the five evaluation methods [12]. ABCDE rule is the most commonly accepted evaluation method for malignancy.

In 1985 the ABCD criteria was established as a simple tool for alerting lay persons and primary health care doctors and to help them diagnose the early incidence of potentially curable melanoma. It consists of a series of simple parameters that can be employed in daily life as a simple mnemonic to make people, as well as doctors, aware of the clinical features of melanoma.

In the mnemonic ABCD; A stands for asymmetry, B stands for border irregularity, C for color variations and D for diameter greater than 6 mm. Asymmetry, border irregularity, and color variation are all associated with melanoma lesions whose diameter are more than 6 mm. Over the later years this ABCD mnemonic

Table 1 How the features affect TDS

Rule	Score	Weight factor
Asymmetry	0–2	1.3
Border	0–8	0.1
Color	1–6	0.5
Diameter/Dermoscopic Structure	1–5	0.5

as a screening tool has changed with the addition of the parameter E, which recognizes evolving lesions (i.e. lesions that change over time). Thus, the mnemonic now reads ABCDE. The parameter E has been included to emphasize the importance of evolving pigmented lesions in the natural process of melanoma progression.

Each of the criteria in ABCDE is then multiplied by a given weight factor to yield a total dermoscopy score (TDS) [13, 14]. Depending on the TDS, malignancy of a lesion is determined. If TDS is less than 4.75 the lesion is considered as benign. The values of 5.45 or greater are highly suggestive of melanoma and the values between 4.8 and 5.45 are considered as suspicious. Table 1 summarizes ranges for ABCD scores and shows weights for each of the criteria. TDS is calculated as follows:

$$TDS = (A \text{ score} \times 1.3) + (B \text{ score} \times 0.1) + (C \text{ score} \times 0.5) + (D \text{ score} \times 0.5)$$

Notice in Table 1 that Color is the major contributor to the TDS score.

3 Density Based Clustering

Density based spatial clustering of applications with noise (DBSCAN) clustering algorithm, introduced in 1996 [15]. It is generally used for discovering clusters in large spatial databases with noise. Fast density-based lesion detection (FDBLD) [16] algorithm borrows cues from DBSCAN; however, FDBLD removes redundant computations in DBSCAN by selectively picking querying points. FDBLD obtained one of the most accurate results in automated lesion border detection.

In this study, the focus is on FDBLD to further improve accuracy of the algorithm for detecting lesion borders in dermoscopy images. FDBLD is highly depended on pre-processing step. In the pre-processing step the intermeans algorithm is used to create a binary image from dermoscopy image [17]. Since a binary image is used in FDBLD, one of the most important components of ABCDE rule, C (color) is missed. Moreover, FDBLD is heavily dependent on the results of the pre-processing step. If another segmentation technique is used for pre-processing, even for the same image, FDBLD tends to generate different results. Therefore, the primary focus on this study is two-fold: first, removing dependency of FDBLD in the pre-processing step; thus, using color information, and second, improving accuracy of the results. To achieve these, new distance measure (normalized distance) is incorporated in to FDBLD.

In the following section DBSCAN and FDBLD algorithms are introduced. It is followed by normalized distance and updated FDBLD. Finally, the experiments and results section compares normalize distance embedded FDBLD (ND-FDBLD) against FDBLD.

3.1 DBSCAN

Density-based clustering methods group data elements based on density characteristics around them. Unlike the majority of other methods, the noises in data can be found as outliers while some other clustering methods force these noises to be a member of a cluster. DBSCAN is based on the formal notion of density-reachability for k-dimensional points. It is designed to discover clusters of arbitrary shape. If region queries are efficiently supported by spatial index structures, i.e. at least in moderately dimensional spaces, runtime of the algorithm is the order of $O(n \log n)$. Two properties are critical for DBSCAN are as follows:

- All points within the cluster are mutually density-connected
- If a point is density-connected to any point of the cluster, it becomes part of the cluster.

If there is a point that does not belong to any cluster yet, these two properties are tested. According to these properties, the point is determined as a member of a specific cluster or otherwise, marked as an outlier. Outlier means point does not belong to any cluster. Even for DBSCAN, distance or similarity measures have critical importance. Depends on the measure used, clustering results vary significantly.

DBSCAN requires two parameters namely epsilon (ε) and a minimum number of points (MinPts) around ε radius of a point. If a point's ε radius vicinity has MinPts number of points around it, then that point is called a core point. DBSCAN is based on a key idea: to form a new cluster or grow an existing cluster the ε-neighborhood of a point should contain at least a minimum number of points, MinPts. Neighbors of a point P are those points that are close to the point P. The neighborhood of a point is determined by choice of a distance function regarding two points in search space, such as Euclidean space. Searching for ε-neighborhood requires a region query, which is, in 2D, to look for neighboring points in ε-radius around a query point. The major advantage of DBSCAN is that it can follow the arbitrary shapes of the clusters and requires only a distance function and two input parameters: ε and MinPts. A detailed theoretical formulation for DBSCAN is given in [15].

Once the two parameters ε and MinPts are set, DBSCAN starts to cluster data points from an arbitrarily chosen point P. It begins with finding the neighbors of point P in ε-neighborhood, i.e., all points that are directly density reachable from point P (see Fig. 2). If the neighborhood is sparsely populated, i.e., it has fewer neighbors than MinPts, point P is labeled as noise. Otherwise, a new cluster is initiated and all points in ε-neighborhood of point P are marked by the new cluster's label. Next, the neighborhoods of all P's neighbors are examined iteratively to check if new candidates can be added into the cluster. If a cluster cannot be expanded further, DBSCAN chooses another arbitrary unlabeled point (if any such point exists)

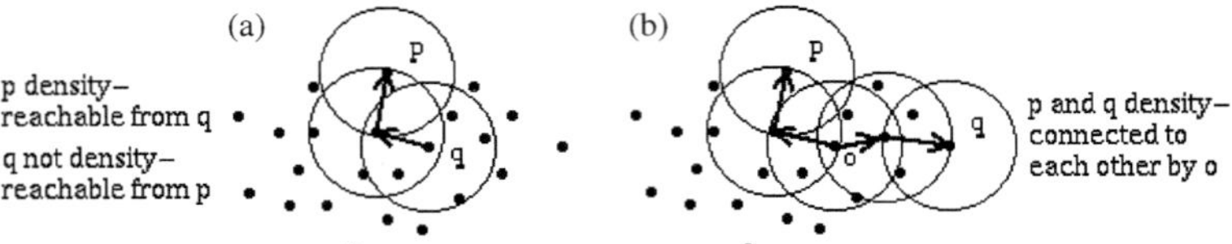

Fig. 2 Density reachability in DBSCAN

and repeats the same procedure to form another cluster. These search-and-create procedures are iterated until all data points in the dataset have been labeled as noise or with a cluster label. The major drawback of DBSCAN is that for a dataset containing n points, n region queries are required to fire during cluster creation.

Regarding a thresholded (binary) image I, let its dimension be $N \times N$. For a pixel p, let p_x and p_y denote its position where top-left corner is $(0, 0)$ of I. Let $c_{xy} = \{0, 1\}$ represent the value of pixel p at (p_x, p_y). Also, let foreground be zero-valued pixels, $c_{xy} = 0$. The ε-neighborhood of a pixel p, denoted by $\text{NEps}(p)$, is defined by

$$\text{NEps}(p) = \{q \in I \mid \text{dist}(p, q) \leq \varepsilon\},$$

where dist() is Euclidean distance, which gives distance between pixels p and q, and given as

$$\text{dist}(p, q) = \sqrt{(p_x - q_x)^2 + (p_y - q_y)^2}.$$

By having $\text{NEps}(p)$, one can create a cluster if $|\text{NEps}(p)| \geq \text{MinPts}$ where and $|\text{NEps}(p)|$ denotes number of ε-neighbors of point p. This final check guarantees that the ε-neighborhood of p is dense enough to form and expand a cluster. As mentioned above, this process continues until all pixels are queried. Finally, noise in dataset (pixels without any cluster label) is assumed not to be part of the foreground.

This clustering algorithm follows the procedure of finding all points density-reachable from an arbitrary starting point. If the starting point is a core point then the procedure begins building a cluster. Recall that, core point is a point which has more than MinPts points around its ε-neighborhood. On the other hand, if the processed point is a border point, the algorithm cannot go further, i.e., DBSCAN cannot find any point density-reachable from the starting point. This procedure is followed until all of the points in the ε-neighborhood are touched or visited at least once. After all of the points in a cluster are visited, the algorithm chooses a new arbitrary starting point to generate other clusters.

3.2 Boundary Driven Density Clustering

DBSCAN spends most of its computational time in region queries. As mentioned in the previous section, the major drawback of DBSCAN for a dataset containing

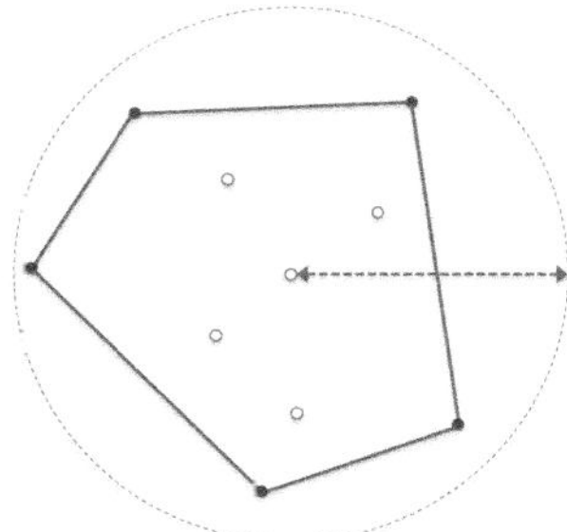

Fig. 3 Convex hull which represents a primitive cluster. MinPts = 5

n points, n region queries are required to complete clustering. Therefore, any improvement in decreasing the number of neighborhood searches will have great impact in terms of the computation time of the algorithm. To this end, FDBLD targets the problem of the excessive number of region queries fired in DBSCAN. For instance, a very large number of region queries become more problematic in the case of applications like virtual slides [18, 19].

Although FDBLD can be generalized for higher dimensional datasets, the applications in 2D are a primary focus of this study. The idea of FDBLD in 2D is to rely on the cluster's boundary. By having these boundaries, it can identify those points that are likely to change current shape, the border of the cluster. In DBSCAN as well as in FDBLD, the area of a cluster always expands out and never shrinks. In the case of queries that cannot affect the cluster's area, looking for the ε-neighborhood is treated as unnecessary and omitted in FDBLD. This improvement certainly is very advantageous for the running time of the algorithm since unnecessary computations are removed. The idea behind determining the border of a cluster is derived from the border of a primitive cluster.

Definition 1 Primitive cluster, PC, is a cluster formed by a core point and bounded by a convex hull.

As seen in Fig. 3, each cluster formation starts with a core point—at the center, which is also the method to create core point candidates. To keep the boundary of a cluster, we represent ε-neighborhood of each core point with a convex hull, which is a special simple polygon. The convex hull encloses all points found in the neighborhood including query at the center.

Figure 4 illustrates how FDBLD works in three steps. In that example assume that a base cluster initially given as in Fig. 4(a). In the first step a core point from border (red point) is queried for $|\text{NEps}(p)| \geq \text{MinPts}$. Assume that MinPts is 5 for this example. So, red point in Fig. 4(a) is a core point. In the second step, a primitive cluster around this center point p is generated with its minimum enclosing convex hull. Notice that, once the ε-neighborhood query is fired around p (red point), we find 8 points (excluding the query point itself) which are more than MinPts of this sample. The convex hull serves as a boundary of PC. PC is shown in Fig. 4(b) (orange convex hull). In the third step, base cluster expanded by merging two polygons;

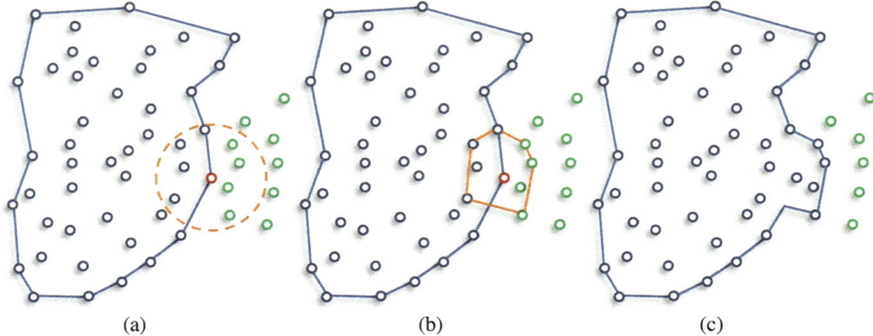

Fig. 4 Expanding a cluster in FDBLD in three steps

base cluster boundary and new convex hull's boundary. Since a cluster never shrinks, it will always expand from border or will remain the same size. This novel idea is called boundary driven density clustering. Interior points are skipped since they cannot expand the current cluster. Therefore, redundant computations in DBSCAN are eliminated; so that, clustering process is accelerated.

Including convex hull in the algorithm accelerates the process and therefore plays an important role. FDBLD also uses monotone chain algorithm [20] to find minimum enclosing convex hull.

3.3 Expanding Cluster in FDBLD

Clustering involves the expansion of the first PC (see Definition 1). Once the first core point in the dataset forms a convex hull it becomes an initial boundary of a cluster. Afterward, each of the convex hulls of core points is combined with main body of the cluster. Principally, this operation corresponds to the union of two polygons.

Adding a convex area can expand the cluster in various ways. Figure 4 shows how a newly found convex hull joins the main body of a cluster in three steps. The ε-neighborhood query (dashed line) in Fig. 4(a) a query (red) point satisfies the MinPts condition; thus, four new points will be added into the existing cluster. The expansion of a cluster iteratively continues by examining other points in the region of leading points until no more unlabeled point is found. The points that are not associated with any cluster are labeled as noise, as it is in DBSCAN.

A simple polygon is the first step in the cluster formation and does not consider donut-like clusters. PCs iteratively form polygon around data points. In Fig. 5(a), assume that PC1 is the first PC formed in the dataset. Since at this time there is no other polygon to be merged, PC1 becomes a polygon at the same time. Once PC2 is obtained, it is unionized with PC1 to expand it. After two more iterations for PC3 and PC4, the final polygon is given in Fig. 5(b). Although one polygon is enough for boundary of a simple cluster (SC), more simple polygons are needed to represent donut-like clusters.

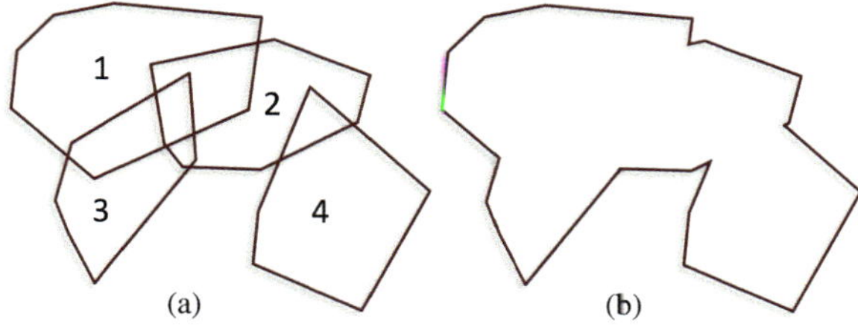

Fig. 5 Unionized convex hulls generate a single polygon

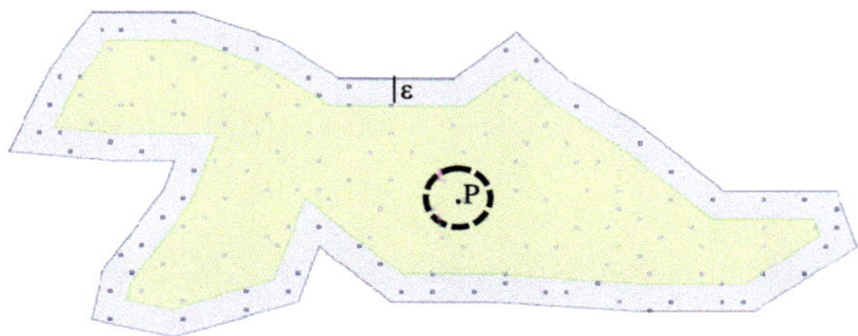

Fig. 6 Leading points (*blue region*)

3.4 Selecting Leading Points

FDBLD differs from DBSCAN in selecting points in order to expand a cluster. Throughout clustering, DBSCAN fires ε-neighborhood query for each point P in a seed list of a growing cluster regardless of its impact on current contours of the cluster. It means that ε-neighborhood queries of the points that cannot alter the boundary of a cluster would waste computational time. Obviously some of the queries would make changes to the shape (see Fig. 6, blue region) while others that are relatively far (ε-width) from the edges would not (see Fig. 6, yellow region). On the other hand, it is important to note that most of the expansions made by a query are not final, and these changes will not be seen in the latest structure of the cluster.

FDBLD only fires queries that potentially change the boundaries of a cluster rather than firing queries for each point in the dataset. That is why FDBLD is a boundary driven density based clustering method. To select leading points, the outlined algorithm keeps the boundaries of the polygons that delineate the cluster body. Accelerations gained with FDBLD compared to DBSCAN are given in Fig. 7. Contrary to DBSCAN, we do not inspect the status of the points, whether they are core or border points, where the label of these points does not have any contributions in terms of the result of clustering. In FDBLD, the cluster body can enlarge only through points that are qualified for an ε-neighborhood queries. Hence, if a point is close enough to a cluster boundary, FDBLD fires ε-neighborhood search around it, otherwise no query will be fired for it. However, it does not mean that every query will alter the shape of a cluster. Therefore, we maintain the set of points (points in the blue region in Fig. 6) that are likely to change the boundaries of a cluster.

As seen in the simple cluster in Fig. 6, the leading data points are only found in the border region (blue region in Fig. 6) including the points on the edges of the outer polygon. The points in the yellow area cannot modify the boundary of a growing

```
Algorithm FDBLD(Binary Image, α, MinPTS)
//BinaryImage is not UNCLASSIFIED
ForeGrd=All zero-value pixels
ClusId = nextId(NOISE);
FOR i FROM 1 TO ForeGrd.size DO
  pxl = ForeGrd.get(i);
  IF pxl.ClId = UNCLASSIFIED THEN
    IF Expand(ForeGrd,pxl,ClusId,α,MinPts) THEN
      ClusId = nextId(ClusId);
    END IF
  END IF
END FOR
END; // FDBLD
```

Fig. 7 Algorithm FDBLD

cluster due to the ε-neighborhood. For instance, point P and its ε-neighborhood dashed circle of Fig. 6 cannot alter the boundary of the cluster; thus, this query will be skipped in FDBLD. Actually, all of the queries for the points in the yellow region in Fig. 6 will be skipped since they cannot alter the cluster. For this reason, the region of leading points, which includes all leading points, can be imagined as an ε-width inner band (blue region Fig. 6) around the polygon of the cluster C.

3.5 FDBLD Algorithm

The algorithm of FDBLD in 2D is given in Fig. 7. Output is the number of clusters found in the image. The major function of FDBLD is Expand which is given in Fig. 8. The boundary of each cluster is obtained from Cls variable, which includes at least one simple polygon.

By firing an ε-neighborhood query around Pxl, CxHull calculates the boundary of Primitive Cluster, PriCls. If the first PriCls is a null pointer structure, Expand returns false for this query pixel. Otherwise, the cluster Cls is formed from PriCls. The next step is to expand as long as the list of boundary pixels is not empty. Union reshapes the current Cls by unionizing PriCls and Cls. Finally, update functions take a list of boundary pixels and current cluster Cls, and return updated boundary pixels. Usually many of pixels are removed from the list because of expansion of the Cls.

In summary, FDBLD was introduced to detect borders of 2D datasets. It is a specialized version of DBSCAN. Although it produces the same clusters as DBSCAN does for the same datasets, on average FDBLD is almost 9 times faster than DBSCAN. In our experiments on 100 dermoscopy images, FDBLD fired 86 % less queries than DBSCAN (see Fig. 9 for comparisons). However, both DBSCAN and FDBLD only work with binary images. Because both of these algorithms necessitate two parameters, ε and MinPts. Without color image to binary image conversion, it was impractical to find a common ε value which fits for all dermoscopy images. Even for our 100 dermoscopy image dataset, it was not possible to find a single ε

```
Boolean Expand(ForeGrd, Pxl, ClusId, α, MinPts)
PriCls = CxHull(Pxl, α, MinPts); //First Pri.Cls.
IF PriCls.size = 0 RETURN FALSE;
ELSE // Core point, PriCls becomes Cls
  Cls = PriCls // Cls is a regular cluster
  Update(BoundPxl,Cls);
  WHILE BoundPxl.size > 0
    Pxl = BoundPxl.next();
    PriCls = CxHull(Pxl, α, MinPts);
    Union(PriCls,Cls);
    Update(BoundPxl,Cls);
  END WHILE; //
END IF
RETURN True;
```

Fig. 8 Expand function for FDBLD

Fig. 9 Number of queries fired by DBSCAN and FDBLD for 100 images

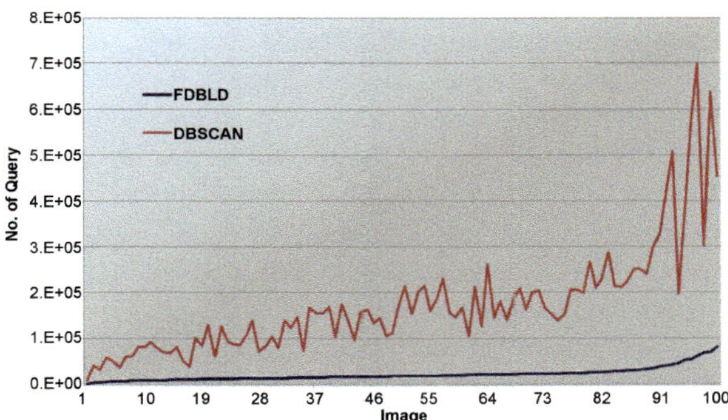

value that produces accurate border regions for all images. This is because each human has almost unique skin color and lesion pigmentations. In order to have single values for ε and MinPts for all images, as an input, both DBSCAN and FDBLD require binary image produced in preprocessing step. When a binary image has been used with DBSCAN or FDBLD; however, very important information, color, is lost.

Recall from the ABCDE Rule section above, in TDS score, color is the most important component for diagnosis. However, both DBSCAN and FDBLD only work with black and white image. To overcome this problem and let FDBLD directly work on a color image without a need for preprocessing step, a new distance measure is necessary. This distance measure should consider both pixel color and position to calculate distance between two pixels. Thus, we developed a new distance measure which is called normalized distance. Normalized distance will be explained in later section. There are many different color spaces. Some of them better fits for certain application area. Thus, normalized distance measure has to be generalized for different color spaces too.

4 Normalized Distance

In this section, a modified normalized distance measure in Euclidean space, which also includes spatial properties of points (pixels in this case), is proposed. The following is a proposed modified normalized distance measure for RGB color space and pixel coordinates:

$$d(i, j) = \sqrt{\frac{w_3(\Delta R)^2 + w_4(\Delta G)^2 + w_5(\Delta B)^2}{3w_1 255^2} + \frac{(\Delta x)^2 + (\Delta y)^2}{w_2((\omega - 1)^2 + (h - 1)^2)}}$$

where $d(i, j)$ represents normalized Euclidean distance between pixels i and j. In the equation, w_3, w_4, and w_5 are weights for individual R, G, and B channels respectively, where initially $w_3 = w_4 = w_5 = 1$. We introduce different weights for different color channels (for future use) since in some application domains certain color channels have more significant impact than others. However, w_1 is weight for RGB color channels against (x, y) coordinates and w_2 is weight for (x, y) coordinates for pixels against RGB color channels, where $1/w1 + 1/w_2 = 1$, by default $w_1 = w_2$. For instance, in some cases if spatial position (x, y coordinate) is more important than color information, then w_1 should be greater than w_2. In that case, the difference in pixel positions will have a greater impact on distance calculation. ΔR, ΔG, ΔB, Δx, and Δy represent RGB channel differences and x, y spatial coordinate differences between two pixels, respectively. 3×255 is RGB channel normalization constant. ω is width and h is height of image for normalization of spatial distance $(\Delta x^2 + \Delta y^2)$.

If we generalize the modified normalized distance measure for different color spaces, it becomes as following:

$$d(i, j) = \sqrt{\frac{\sum_{k=1}^{n} w_{k+2}(\Delta C_k)^2}{n w_1 C_{\max}^2} + \frac{(\Delta x)^2 + (\Delta y)^2}{w_2((\omega - 1)^2 + (h - 1)^2)}}$$

where k is the multispectral channel number, n is the total number of channels, ΔC_k represents channel k's difference between i and j, w_k represents weights for each channel where $\sum_{k=1}^{n} w_{k+2} = 1$. In this way, both color and spatial position information are included in a single distance metric. With this distance measure, it becomes possible to differentiate the same colored pixels in different locations.

Figure 10 illustrates the importance of normalized distance measure over results: (a) shows an exemplary dermoscopy image of a lesion which has low contrast between the surrounding skin and the lesion and also a fuzzy and irregular le sion border; (b) illustrates the result drawn by a dermatologist whereas (c) illustrates the result generated by FDBLD with Manhattan distance while (d) illustrates the result generated by ND-FDBLD. As clearly seen from this example, the simple normalized distance measure was specifically designed for lesion border detections (ND-FDBLD) outperform FDBLD. (e) shows the result of FDBLD with Euclidean distance (after preprocessing is applied). (f) and (g) illustrate how ND-FDBLD behaves with different weights. Moreover, normalized distance (ND) makes a finding common ε value for all images very simple. ε interval is found in a few trials. With

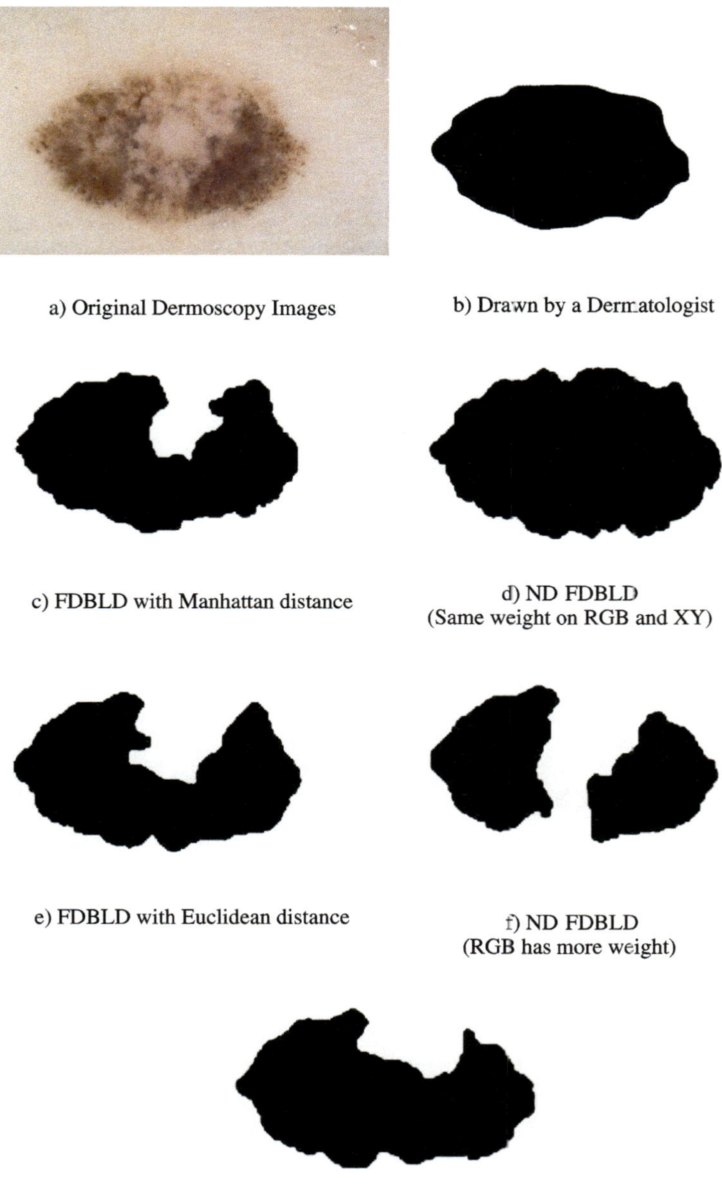

a) Original Dermoscopy Images

b) Drawn by a Dermatologist

c) FDBLD with Manhattan distance

d) ND FDBLD
(Same weight on RGB and XY)

e) FDBLD with Euclidean distance

f) ND FDBLD
(RGB has more weight)

g) ND FDBLD (XY has more weight)

Fig. 10 Results generated by FDBLD with different distance measures

FDBLD without pre-processing, it is not possible to find common ε interval which generates satisfactory results for all images. ND-FDBLD works directly on color images without any pre-processing (intermeans segmentation) step.

4.1 Effect of Color Spaces

Although ND benefits this study in RGB space, it is adaptable to other space. The weights w_i are, therefore, incorporated into the calculation of ND. Note that color is represented differently in different color space. In majority of biomedical applications, color is the most critical information for assessing biomedical images. However, in literature, there is no standard color space in which a particular color points are represented for computer vision tasks.

A standard language within the community to quantify and collaborate is a much needed effort. In 1931, an international group, Commission Internationale de L'Eclairage[1] (CIE), had met to bring a solution to the mentioned difficulty. This effort resulted in a very useful tool: color models, which is the fundamental brick for people and devices to work and communicate in agreement while using digital color images. The naming of a color model allows quantifying colors that remove subjectivity.

A color model provides a coordinate system and a subspace in which each color is represented by a single point. Beside generic color models, many commercial models, such as Munsell [21], Hunter-LAB [22], TexHVC and NCS [23], were also invented for various applications. In the digital image processing, there are more than 20 well-accepted color models. For instance, CIELAB, CIELUV, CIEXYZ, CMY, CMYK, HSL, HSV, Hunter-LAB, NRGB, RGB, and SCT are the most common color models. A few of them are used extensively, whereas others appear only in a few studies. Most of the researchers [19, 24–26] map their color points to another color space in the preprocessing phase. It is often claimed that mapping will benefit the general framework, such as CBIR, classification of subimages, and texture analysis. One of the expected advantages of conversion between color models is to have perceptual uniformity in the new color space [24]. Perceptual uniformity is an attribute of color space, and characterizes a just-detectable visual difference that constitutes a constant distance (such as Euclidean) in any location or direction within the space [25]. More formally, considering the distance from $C1 = (X1, Y1, Z1)$ to color $C1 + \Delta C$, and the distance from color $C2 = (X2, Y2, Z2)$ to color $C2 + \Delta C$, where $\Delta C = (\Delta X, \Delta Y, \Delta Z)$. Both distances are equal to ΔC, yet in general, they will not be perceived as being equal colors by human eye. This is because of the variation throughout the spectrum of color models. CIELAB and CIELUV were particularly design to overcome this problem. Reader is referred to [26, 27] for details on analysis of color models on biomedical image processing.

---

[1]This is also called the International Commission on Illumination.

5 Experiments and Results on Dermoscopy Images

Initially, we studied on FDBLD clustering algorithm to find the two main parameters, MinPts and ε. An empirical experimentation was employed to determine these two parameters. We randomly selected 50 dermoscopy images in order to find the correct values for MinPts and ε. After the parameters are determined, new ND embedded FDBLD is tested on 100 dermoscopy images. Tables 2 and 3 illustrate the difference between ND-based FDBLD and FDBLD of Mete et al. [16]. The first column of a table is image ID's of 100 dermoscopy images. Each object in an image is labeled after applying the clustering algorithm. The results essentially indicate two labels: cancer and non-cancer. In this comparison, precision, recall, and border error are used. We calculated these measurements by using the formula below.

$$Precision = \frac{TP}{TP + FP}, \quad \text{and} \quad Recall = \frac{TP}{TP + FN}$$

Border error (BE) measure, which is also called XOR measure, was proposed by Hance et al. [28]. This measure quantifies the percentage of border detection error. It is the most commonly used measure and accepted by the skin lesion detection researchers. Thus, XOR measure is more important for skin lesion detection than precision and recall. Schaefer et al. [29] also uses XOR measure for dermoscopy images, and it is calculated by

$$BE = \left[\frac{AB \oplus MB}{MB} \right] \times 100$$

where $\oplus$ is exclusive OR operator, essentially underlines disagreement between the target (ManualBorder, MB) and predicted (Automatic Border, AB) regions. Refer-

Table 2 Comparisons between ND-FDBLD and FDBLD with respect to border error rate, precision, and recall (first half of the dataset)

Img.ID	ND-FDBLD			FDBLD		
	B. Err.	Pre.	Rec.	B. Err.	Pre.	Rec.
1	0.05	0.96	0.99	0.03	1.00	0.88
2	0.08	0.92	0.98	0.02	0.94	0.86
3	0.08	0.96	0.96	0.09	0.89	0.76
4	0.04	0.97	1.00	0.08	0.98	0.79
5	0.06	0.95	0.99	0.04	1.00	0.76
6	0.04	0.98	0.98	0.05	0.98	0.86
7	0.06	0.95	0.99	0.08	0.93	0.87
8	0.04	0.96	1.00	0.05	0.89	0.85
9	0.04	0.97	0.98	0.06	1.00	0.84
10	0.06	0.94	1.00	0.06	1.00	0.86
11	0.10	0.91	1.00	0.04	1.00	0.84
12	0.03	0.98	1.00	0.04	0.96	0.89

Table 2 (Continued)

Img.ID	ND-FDBLD			FDBLD		
	B. Err.	Pre.	Rec.	B. Err.	Pre.	Rec.
13	0.04	0.96	1.00	0.03	1.00	0.88
14	0.08	0.93	1.00	0.03	1.00	0.85
15	0.02	0.98	0.99	0.02	1.00	0.93
16	0.01	1.00	0.99	0.01	0.99	0.94
17	0.06	0.94	1.00	0.08	1.00	0.57
18	0.06	0.96	0.98	0.11	1.00	0.68
19	0.13	0.89	1.00	0.13	1.00	0.72
20	0.02	1.00	0.98	0.05	1.00	0.71
21	0.03	0.99	0.98	0.05	1.00	0.80
22	0.01	0.99	0.99	0.04	1.00	0.76
23	0.02	0.99	0.99	0.04	1.00	0.85
24	0.02	0.98	1.00	0.06	1.00	0.71
25	0.03	1.00	0.97	0.05	1.00	0.87
26	0.04	1.00	0.97	0.05	1.00	0.85
27	0.04	0.97	0.98	0.07	1.00	0.82
28	0.03	0.99	0.99	0.06	1.00	0.82
29	0.05	0.96	0.99	0.07	1.00	0.76
30	0.02	0.98	1.00	0.05	1.00	0.80
31	0.33	0.75	1.00	0.33	1.00	0.52
32	0.04	0.96	1.00	0.08	1.00	0.76
33	0.06	0.94	1.00	0.06	1.00	0.70
34	0.04	0.97	0.99	0.08	1.00	0.79
35	0.05	0.98	0.97	0.06	1.00	0.83
36	0.11	0.90	1.00	0.07	1.00	0.77
37	0.03	0.98	1.00	0.09	1.00	0.80
38	0.04	0.96	1.00	0.02	0.99	0.90
39	0.03	0.98	0.99	0.03	1.00	0.90
40	0.01	1.00	0.99	0.02	1.00	0.92
41	0.03	0.99	0.97	0.05	1.00	0.82
42	0.02	1.00	0.98	0.03	1.00	0.88
43	0.02	1.00	0.98	0.06	1.00	0.76
44	0.04	1.00	0.96	0.02	1.00	0.86
45	0.01	0.99	1.00	0.04	1.00	0.82
46	0.04	0.96	1.00	0.08	1.00	0.73
47	0.02	1.00	0.98	0.03	1.00	0.85
48	0.04	0.97	1.00	0.08	1.00	0.73
49	0.05	0.96	1.00	0.15	1.00	0.73
50	0.01	0.99	1.00	0.04	1.00	0.83

Table 3 Comparisons between ND-FDBLD and FDBLD with respect to border error rate, precision, and recall (second half of the dataset)

Img.ID	ND-FDBLD			FDBLD		
	B. Err.	Pre.	Rec.	B. Err.	Pre.	Rec.
51	0.09	1.00	0.91	0.03	1.00	0.93
52	0.08	1.00	0.92	0.05	1.00	0.83
53	0.04	1.00	0.96	0.02	0.99	0.90
54	0.04	0.97	1.00	0.09	1.00	0.73
55	0.05	0.96	1.00	0.08	1.00	0.75
56	0.03	0.99	0.97	0.05	1.00	0.81
57	0.05	1.00	0.95	0.06	1.00	0.83
58	0.03	1.00	0.97	0.05	1.00	0.83
59	0.05	1.00	0.95	0.01	1.00	0.96
60	0.05	0.98	0.97	0.03	1.00	0.91
61	0.06	0.95	1.00	0.14	1.00	0.62
62	0.03	0.99	0.98	0.07	1.00	0.81
63	0.02	0.98	0.99	0.06	1.00	0.81
64	0.03	1.00	0.97	0.03	1.00	0.81
65	0.01	1.00	0.99	0.01	1.00	0.92
66	0.02	0.99	1.00	0.05	0.90	0.80
67	0.03	0.97	1.00	0.05	1.00	0.77
68	0.02	0.98	1.00	0.04	1.00	0.81
69	0.01	1.00	0.99	0.01	1.00	0.90
70	0.03	1.00	0.97	0.02	1.00	0.80
71	0.03	0.98	0.99	0.06	1.00	0.68
72	0.04	0.96	1.00	0.10	1.00	0.68
73	0.05	0.99	0.96	0.05	0.94	0.77
74	0.01	0.99	1.00	0.02	0.99	0.85
75	0.07	0.94	1.00	0.08	1.00	0.65
76	0.40	0.72	1.00	0.11	1.00	0.71
77	0.01	0.99	1.00	0.03	1.00	0.73
78	0.11	0.90	1.00	0.13	1.00	0.62
79	0.14	0.88	1.00	0.12	1.00	0.69
80	0.04	0.96	1.00	0.07	1.00	0.63
81	0.01	1.00	1.00	0.02	1.00	0.61
82	0.14	0.88	1.00	0.12	1.00	0.74
83	0.05	0.96	1.00	0.11	1.00	0.52
84	0.01	0.99	1.00	0.03	1.00	0.78
85	0.04	0.97	0.99	0.08	1.00	0.76
86	0.05	0.98	0.97	0.09	0.98	0.76
87	0.03	0.98	0.99	0.07	1.00	0.73

Table 3 (Continued)

Img.ID	ND-FDBLD			FDBLD		
	B. Err.	Pre.	Rec.	B. Err.	Pre.	Rec.
88	0.02	0.98	1.00	0.06	1.00	0.55
89	0.03	0.99	0.98	0.04	0.89	0.90
90	0.07	0.95	0.98	0.17	1.00	0.55
91	0.03	0.97	1.00	0.08	1.00	0.61
92	0.06	0.97	0.98	0.05	1.00	0.88
93	0.02	0.98	1.00	0.02	1.00	0.90
94	0.06	0.96	0.98	0.15	1.00	0.65
95	0.01	1.00	0.99	0.03	1.00	0.66
96	0.06	0.98	0.96	0.09	1.00	0.74
97	0.31	0.76	1.00	0.23	1.00	0.65
98	0.04	0.96	0.99	0.05	1.00	0.83
99	0.05	0.95	1.00	0.12	1.00	0.64
100	0.03	0.97	1.00	0.03	1.00	0.70

ring to information retrieval terminology, the nominator of the *BE* means summation of false positive (*FP*) and false negative (*FN*). The denominator is obtained by adding true positive (*TP*) to false negatives (*FN*). After the pixels in an image are labeled, the number of true prediction of the lesion area was named true positive, the number of false prediction of lesion area as false positive, the number of true prediction of non-lesion as true negative, and the number of false prediction of non-lesion as false negative.

Of 100 images, in 75 images ND-FDBLD had better results than FDBLD (see Fig. 10). In Tables 2 and 3, ND-FDBLD is compared against the original FDBLD on the same dataset. The three columns following the first column show our results and the second three columns represent results from Mete et al. [16].

As seen from Tables 2 and 3, the proposed lesion border detection method is more accurate than FDBLD. However, FDBLD outperforms our method in two images, image numbers 76 and 97 (Fig. 11). In these images, there exists a cutaneous feature which is hair. In these images, hair occludes the lesion area and they elongate down to the image borders which are considered as peripherals in our approach. Therefore, hairs which intersect the lesion area and the regions residing between the hairs are included in the lesion area. An active contour model introduced recently overcomes this problem [30].

6 Conclusion

A recent study of the fast density based lesion border detection (FDBLD) approach. Reference [16] was used as a basis for this study. FDBLD is based on a novel boundary driven density based clustering algorithm. FDBLD as well as its predecessor

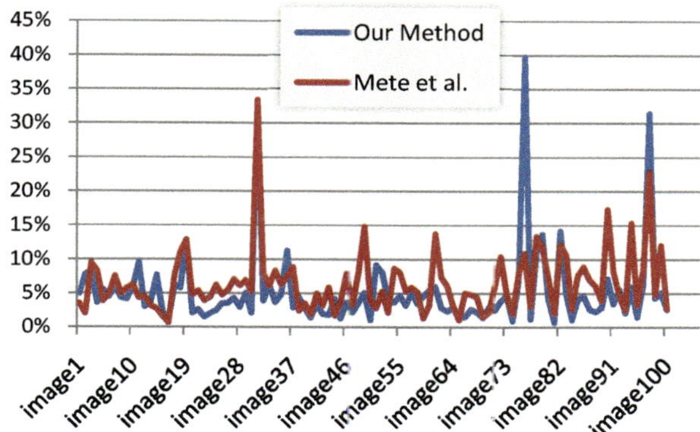

Fig. 11 Comparison between our method and FDBLD, x horizontal axes is image numbers, vertical one is border error of corresponding image

DBSCAN requires two parameters ε and MinPts. To find optimum parameters for ε and MinPts that fit for every image in our dermoscopy dataset is not possible. Thus, FDBLD has to have binary image. When it runs on a binary image; however, the most important component of dermoscopy image, color, is lost. In this study, to overcome this problem and eliminate pre-processing step (color to binary image conversion), we introduce a new distance measure. This distance measure is called normalized distance (ND). ND not only considers pixel positions but also considers pixel colors for distance computation. Moreover, ND is generalized to fit other color spaces than RGB.

Accuracy of the FDBLD is highly dependent on the preprocessing step. To improve accuracy of the FDBLD, to remove its dependency on the preprocessing step, and to let FDBLD directly run on color dermoscopy images ND is integrated to the existing approach. ND integrated FDBLD is abbreviated as ND-FDBLD.

Results show that dependency of FDBLD to the pre-processing step is discarded by integrating normalized distance measure in to FDBLD. Moreover, efficiency of the FDBLD is improved by achieving lower border error rates for automated lesion border detections in dermoscopy images. ND-FDBLD was tested on 100 dermoscopy images. Results were compared with both FDBLD and manually drawn lesion borders by dermatologists for the same images. In order to measure accuracy of the obtained results, precision, recall, and border error rate measures were used. The results show that ND-FDBLD performs better in 75 % of dermoscopy images than FDBLD. Moreover, this new approach reduces overall border error rates. Future direction includes noise reduction in the preprocessing steps and finding the best color space for dermoscopic image analysis.

Acknowledgements This study is partially supported by University Research Council at University of Central Arkansas. Part of this research is funded by Graduate School of TAMU-Commerce.

References

1. AmericanCancerSociety (2010) Cancer facts & figures. Available: http://www.cancer.org/acs/groups/content/@nho/documents/document/acspc-024113.pdf

2. Jemal A, Siegel R, Xu J, Ward E (2010) Cancer statistics, 2010. CA Cancer J Clin 60:277–300
3. Rigel DS, Carucci JA (2000) Malignant melanoma: prevention, early detection, and treatment in the 21st century. CA Cancer J Clin 50:215–236
4. Binder M, Schwarz M, Winkler A, Steiner A, Kaider A, Wolff K, Pehamberger H (1995) Epiluminescence microscopy. A useful tool for the diagnosis of pigmented skin lesions for formally trained dermatologists. Arch Dermatol 131:286–291
5. Celebi ME, Iyatomi H, Schaefer G, Stoecker WV (2009) Lesion border detection in dermoscopy images. Comput Med Imaging Graph 33:148–153
6. Emre Celebi M, Alp Aslandogan Y, Stoecker WV, Iyatomi H, Oka H, Chen X (2007) Unsupervised border detection in dermoscopy images. Skin Res Technol 13:454–462
7. Pratt WK (2007) Digital image processing: PIKS scientific inside, 4th edn. Wiley-Interscience, Hoboken
8. Celebi ME, Wen Q, Hwang S, Iyatomi H, Schaefer G (2012) Lesion border detection in dermoscopy images using ensembles of thresholding methods. Skin Res Technol (in press)
9. Gomez DD, Butakoff C, Ersboll BK, Stoecker W (2008) Independent histogram pursuit for segmentation of skin lesions. IEEE Trans Biomed Eng 55:157–161
10. Celebi ME, Kingravi HA, Iyatomi H, Aslandogan YA, Stoecker WV, Moss RH, Malters JM, Grichnik JM, Marghoob AA, Rabinovitz HS, Menzies SW (2008) Border detection in dermoscopy images using statistical region merging. Skin Res Technol 14:347–353
11. Sonka M, Hlavac V, Boyle R (1999) Image processing, analysis, and machine vision, vol 2. PWS, Pacific Grove
12. Argenziano G, Soyer HP, Chimenti S, Talamini R, Corona R, Sera F, Binder M, Cerroni L, De Rosa G, Ferrara G (2003) Dermoscopy of pigmented skin lesions: results of a consensus meeting via the Internet. J Am Acad Dermatol 48:679–693
13. Nachbar F, Stolz W, Merkle T, Cognetta AB, Vogt T, Landthaler M, Bilek P, Braun-Falco O, Plewig G (1994) The ABCD rule of dermatoscopy. High prospective value in the diagnosis of doubtful melanocytic skin lesions. J Am Acad Dermatol 30:551–559
14. Argenziano G, Fabbrocini G, Carli P, De Giorgi V, Sammarco E, Delfino M (1998) Epiluminescence microscopy for the diagnosis of doubtful melanocytic skin lesions. Comparison of the ABCD rule of dermatoscopy and a new 7-point checklist based on pattern analysis. Arch Dermatol 134:1563–1570
15. Ester M, Kriegel HP, Sander J, Xu X (1996) A density-based algorithm for discovering clusters in large spatial databases with noise. In: Proceedings of KDD, pp 226–231
16. Mete M, Kockara S, Aydin K (2011) Fast density-based lesion detection in dermoscopy images. Comput Med Imaging Graph 35:128–136
17. Otsu N (1979) A threshold selection method from gray-level histograms. IEEE Trans Syst Man Cybern 9:62–66
18. Sertel O, Kong J, Shimada H, Catalyurek U, Saltz JH, Gurcan MN (2009) Computer-aided prognosis of neuroblastoma on whole-slide images: classification of stromal development. Pattern Recognit 42:1093–1103
19. Mete M, Hennings L, Spencer HJ, Topaloglu U (2009) Automatic identification of angiogenesis in double stained images of liver tissue. BMC Bioinform 10(Suppl 11):S13
20. Andrew A (1979) Another efficient algorithm for convex hulls in two dimensions. Inf Process Lett 9:216–219
21. Cleland TM (2004) A practical description of the munsell color system and suggestions for its use 1937. Kessinger Publishing, LLC, Baltimore
22. Hunter RS (1948) Minutes of the thirty-first meeting of the board of directors of the optical society of America, incorporated. J Opt Soc Am 38:651
23. Hård A, Sivik L (1981) NCS—natural color system: a Swedish standard for color notation. Color Res Appl 6:129–138
24. Umbaugh SE (2005) Computer imaging: digital image analysis and processing. CRC, Boca Raton
25. Russ JC (2007) The image processing handbook. CRC, Boca Raton

26. Mete M, Topaloglu U (2009) Statistical comparison of color model-classifier pairs in hematoxylin and eosin stained histological images. In: Proceedings of the IEEE symposium on computational intelligence in bioinformatics and computational biology, pp 284–291
27. Celebi ME, Kingravi HA, Celiker F (2010) Fast colour space transformations using minimax approximations. IET Image Process 4:70–80
28. Hance GA, Umbaugh SE, Moss RH, Stoecker WV (1996) Unsupervised color image segmentation: with application to skin tumor borders. IEEE Eng Med Biol Mag 15:104–111
29. Schaefer G, Rajab MI, Emre Celebi M, Iyatomi H (2011) Colour and contrast enhancement for improved skin lesion segmentation. Comput Med Imaging Graph 35:99–104
30. Mete M, Sirakov NM (2010) Lesion detection in demoscopy images with novel density-based and active contour approaches. BMC Bioinform 11:S23

A Color and Texture Based Hierarchical K-NN Approach to the Classification of Non-melanoma Skin Lesions

Lucia Ballerini, Robert B. Fisher, Ben Aldridge, and Jonathan Rees

Abstract This chapter proposes a novel hierarchical classification system based on the K-Nearest Neighbors (K-NN) model and its application to non-melanoma skin lesion classification. Color and texture features are extracted from skin lesion images. The hierarchical structure decomposes the classification task into a set of simpler problems, one at each node of the classification. Feature selection is embedded in the hierarchical framework that chooses the most relevant feature subsets at each node of the hierarchy. The accuracy of the proposed hierarchical scheme is higher than 93 % in discriminating cancer and potential at risk lesions from benign lesions, and it reaches an overall classification accuracy of 74 % over five common classes of skin lesions, including two non-melanoma cancer types. This is the most extensive known result on non-melanoma skin cancer classification using color and texture information from images acquired by a standard camera (non-dermoscopy).

1 Introduction

Skin cancers are the most common forms of human malignancies in fair skinned populations [18]. Although malignant melanoma is the form of "skin cancer" with the highest mortality, the "non-melanoma skin cancers" (basal cell carcinomas and squamous cell carcinomas, etc.) are far more common. The incidence of both melanoma and non-melanoma skin cancers is increasing, with the number of cases

L. Ballerini (✉) · R.B. Fisher
School of Informatics, University of Edinburgh, Edinburgh, UK
e-mail: lucia.ballerini@ed.ac.uk

R.B. Fisher
e-mail: rbf@inf.ed.ac.uk

B. Aldridge · J. Rees
Department of Dermatology, University of Edinburgh, Edinburgh UK

B. Aldridge
e-mail: ben.aldridge@ed.ac.uk

J. Rees
e-mail: jonathan.rees@ed.ac.uk

M.E. Celebi, G. Schaefer (eds.), *Color Medical Image Analysis*,
Lecture Notes in Computational Vision and Biomechanics 6,
DOI 10.1007/978-94-007-5389-1_4, © Springer Science+Business Media Dordrecht 2013

being diagnosed doubling approximately every 15 years [35]. It is widely accepted that early detection is fundamental to reducing the diseases' morbidity and mortality. Automatic detection systems may offer benefit for this key diagnostic task.

There are a considerable number of published studies on classification methods relating to the diagnosis of cutaneous malignancies. The first published work presenting an automatic classification of melanoma could be found in 1987 [11]. A paper describing the first complete system appeared a few years later [29]. The number of published papers has increased every year and the significant progress that has occurred in this field is demonstrated by the recent journal special issue that summarizes the state of the art in computerized analysis of skin cancer images and provides future directions for this exciting subfield of medical image analysis [16].

Different techniques for enhancement, segmentation, feature extraction and classification have been reported by several authors. Enhancement includes color calibration and normalization [32, 54].

Concerning segmentation, Celebi et al. [14] presented a systematic overview of main border detection methods: clustering followed by active contours are the most popular. Improvements in lesion border detection are described in recent papers [26, 39, 54, 61, 66].

Numerous features have been extracted from skin images, including shape, color, texture and border properties [19, 37, 43, 52, 56, 57, 63]. It is common to use features related to the ABCD mnemonic rule [49]. However, our experiments suggested that the use of the ABCD rule in the development of automatic classifiers can be arguably discouraged [64].

Classification methods range from discriminant analysis to neural networks and support vector machines [15, 41, 55]. See Maglogiannis et al. [40] for a review of the state of the art of computer vision system for skin lesion characterization.

These methods have been mainly developed for images acquired by epiluminescence microscopy (ELM or dermoscopy). However, newer technologies, including digital dermoscopy, infrared imaging, multispectral imaging, and confocal microscopy, have recently come to the forefront in providing greater diagnostic accuracy [16].

Moreover published studies mainly focus on differentiating melanocytic naevi (moles) from melanoma. Whilst this is undeniably important (as malignant melanoma is the form of skin cancer with the highest mortality), in the "real-world" the majority of lesions presenting to dermatologists for assessment are not covered by this narrow domain, and such systems ignore other benign lesions and crucially the two most common skin cancers (Squamous Cell Carcinomas and Basal Cell Carcinomas) [10, 27, 60].

The proposed work uses only high resolution color images acquired using standard cameras. To our knowledge only two melanoma pre-screening systems are based on standard camera images [1, 12].

In the current study, color and texture features are used for the classification. We focus on 5 common classes of skin lesions: Actinic Keratosis (AK), Basal Cell Carcinoma (BCC), Melanocytic Nevus/Mole (ML), Squamous Cell Carcinoma (SCC), Seborrhoeic Keratosis (SK). As far as we can tell there is no research on automatic classification of these lesion types (other than moles) outside our group [39].

Moreover, this paper introduces a new hierarchical framework for skin lesion classification. This framework is comprised of a modified version of the K-Nearest Neighbors (K-NN) classifier, the Hierarchical K-Nearest Neighbors (HKNN) classifier, and a new similarity measure, based on color and texture features, that uses different feature sets for comparing similarity at each node of the hierarchy.

The motivation for using a K-NN classifier can be seen in Fig. 4. It is clear that the clusters overlap greatly, but are distinguishable. No hard boundary could separate them (e.g. as usable by a support vector machine or Bayesian classifier).

Below we describe how the lesion classes can be organized in a hierarchical scheme (Sect. 2) that suggests the use of the hierarchical classifier (Sect. 3). Then we introduce the feature pool (Sect. 4). Therefore we make 2 claims:

1. The use of a hierarchical K-NN classifier improves classification accuracy from 70 % to 74 % over a non-hierarchical K-NN, and from 67 % and 69 % over a flat and a hierarchical Bayes classifier, respectively,
2. This is the most extensive paper to present lesion classification results for non-melanoma skin cancer using color imagery acquired by a standard camera, unlike the dermoscopy method, which requires a specialised sensor.

While 74 % is low compared to the 90+ % rates achieved by melanoma classification, we argue that 74 % is worth publication: (a) the melanoma results are from only the 2 class problem of melanoma vs melanocytic naevi (moles), and (b) it has taken more than 20 years of research specifically on that problem to reach the 90+ % levels, whereas this is the first research on image-based classification of AK, BCC, SCC and SK. We accept that whilst classification rates of this magnitude seem low in the sphere of informatics research, these rates are significantly above what is currently being achieved in non-specialist medical practice [10, 21, 27, 44, 51, 60].

2 Skin Class Hierarchy

Some images of the five classes are shown in Fig. 1. The hierarchy is fixed *a priori* by grouping our image classes into two main groups. The first group, hence called *Group1*, contains lesion classes: Actinic Keratosis (AK), Basal Cell Carcinoma (BCC) and Squamous Cell Carcinoma (SCC). The second group, hence called *Group2*, contains lesion classes: Melanocytic Nevus/Mole (ML) and Seborrhoeic Keratosis (SK). We note that AK, BCC, SCC, ML and SK are diagnostic classes defined by dermatologists. The two groups were constructed by clustering classes containing images which were visually similar at the first split. However we can give some meaning to two groups observing that the first group comprises BCC and SCC that are the two most common types of skin cancer and AK which is considered a pre-malignant condition that can give rise to SCCs and sometimes can be visually similar to early superficial BCCs. In the second group ML and SK are both benign forms of skin lesions having a similar appearance. The class grouping leads to the hierarchical structure shown in Fig. 2. This structure makes a coarse separation among classes at the upper level while finer decisions are made at a lower level. As a result, this scheme decomposes the original problem into 3 sub-problems.

Fig. 1 Examples of skin lesion images from the different classes used in this work

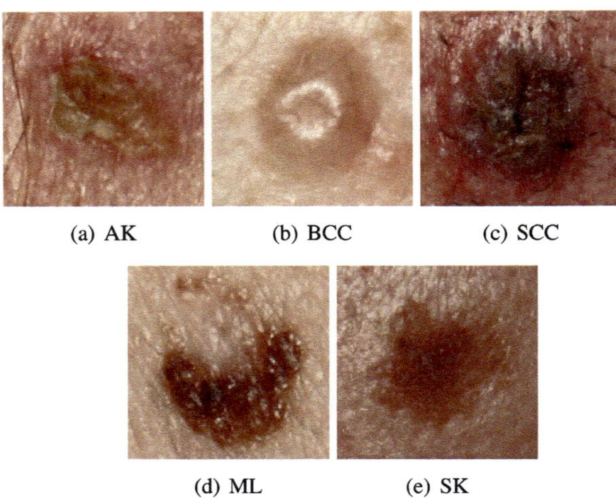

(a) AK   (b) BCC   (c) SCC

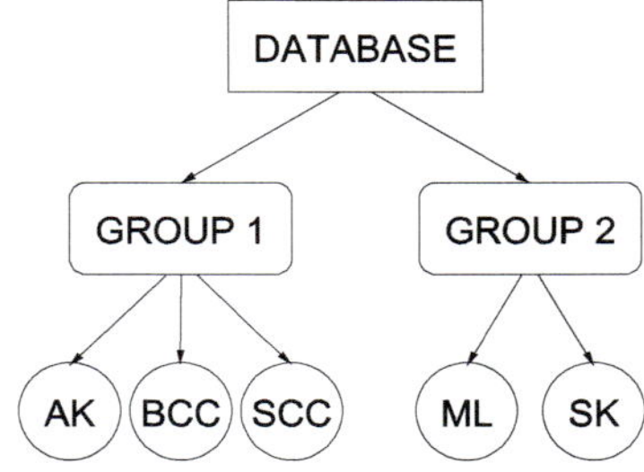

(d) ML   (e) SK

Fig. 2 Block diagram of the hierarchical organization of skin lesion classes

3 Hierarchical K-NN Classifier

A large number of classifier combinations have been proposed in the literature [33]. They may have different feature sets, different training sets, different classification methods or different training sessions, all resulting in a set of classifiers whose output may be combined, with the hope of improving the overall classification accuracy. The schemes for combining multiple classifiers can be grouped into three main categories according to their architecture: (1) parallel, (2) cascading and (3) hierarchical. In the hierarchical architecture, individual classifiers are combined into a structure which is similar to a decision tree classifier. The advantage of this architecture is the high efficiency and flexibility in exploiting the discriminant power of different types of features [33]. A large number of studies have shown that classifier combination can improve recognition accuracy [33]. It has been shown that in many domains an ensemble of classifiers outperforms any of its single components [42]. The approach used in our research falls within the hierarchical model.

Our approach divides the classification task into a set of smaller classification problems corresponding to the splits in the classification hierarchy (see Fig. 2). Each of these subtasks is significantly simpler than the original task, since the classifier at a node in the hierarchy need only distinguish between a smaller number of classes. Therefore, it may be possible to separate the smaller number of classes with higher accuracy. Moreover, it may be possible to make this determination based on a smaller set of features.

The proposed approach addresses also the feature selection problem. The reduction in the feature space avoids many problems related to high dimensional feature spaces, such as the "curse of dimensionality" problem [33], where the indexing structures degrade and the significance of each feature decreases, making the process of storing, indexing and classifying extremely time consuming. Moreover, in several situations, many features are correlated, meaning that they bring redundant information about the images that can deteriorate the ability of the system to correctly distinguish them. Dimensionality reduction or feature selection has been an active research area in pattern recognition, statistics and data mining communities. The main idea of feature selection is to choose a subset of input features by eliminating features with little or no predictive information.

It is important to note that the key here is not merely the use of feature selection, but its integration with the hierarchical structure. In practice we build different classifiers using different sets of training images (according to the set of classifications made at the higher levels of the hierarchy). So each classifier uses a different set of features optimized for those images. This forces the individual classifiers to use potentially independent information.

Hierarchical classifiers are well known [28, 45, 58] and commonly used for document and text classification [13, 20, 23, 50], including a hierarchical K-NN classifier [24]. While we found papers describing applications of hierarchical systems to medical image classification and annotation tasks [22, 47, 59], to the best of our knowledge only a hierarchical neural network model has been applied to skin lesions [53]. They claim over 90 % accuracy on 58 images including 4 melanomas. Unfortunately many technical details are not described in the paper. On the other hand, only poor performance was reported relative to the classification of melanoma using the K-NN method [7, 31]. Some promising results have been presented very recently by using a K-NN followed by a Decision Tree classifier [12].

3.1 K-NN Classifier

K-NN is a well-known classifier. K-NN was first introduced by Fix and Hodges [25] in 1951. It is well explored in the literature and has been shown to have good classification performance on a wide range of real world data sets [17]. Many *lazy learning algorithms* are derivatives of the K-NN. A review of them is presented in the paper of Wetterschereck et al. [62]. A recent application of one of these similarity-based learning algorithms, namely the lazy CL procedure, to melanoma is described by Armengol [5].

To classify an unknown example T, the K-NN classifier finds the K nearest neighbors among the training data and uses the categories of the K neighbors to weight the category candidates. Then majority voting among the categories of data in the neighborhood is used to decide the class label of T. Given M classes $C_1, C_2, \ldots, C_M$ and N training samples $I_1, I_2, \ldots, I_N$, and the classification for I_i with respect to category C_j ($i = 1, \ldots, N; j = 1, \ldots, M$):

$$y(I_i, C_j) = \begin{cases} 1 & I_i \in C_j \\ 0 & I_i \notin C_j \end{cases} \tag{1}$$

the decision rule in K-NN can be written as:

$$\text{assign } T \text{ to } C_j \text{ if } score(T, C_j) = \arg\max_{j=1}^{M} \sum_{i=1}^{K} y(I_i, C_j) \tag{2}$$

where the training examples I_i are ranked according to their similarity to the test example T.

The K-NN classifier has only one free parameter K which can be optimized by a leave-one-out cross-validation procedure, given the distance function $Dist$ (see Eq. (13)) which is used to determine the 'nearest' neighbors. Choosing the properties to be used in each classifier is a core issue, and is addressed next. The actual distance metrics are presented in Sect. 4.

3.2 Learning Phase

Our Hierarchical K-NN classifier (HKNN) is composed of three distinct K-NN classifier systems, one at the top level, and two at the bottom level. The top level classifier is fed with all the images in the training set. It classifies them into one of the two groups. The other two classifiers are trained using only the images of the corresponding group (i.e. AK/BCC/SCC or ML/SK) that have been correctly (when in the training stage) classified by the top classifier, and classifies them into one of the 2 or 3 diagnostic classes.

The learning phase consists of the feature selection process for the three distinct K-NN classifiers. A sequential forward selection algorithm [34] (SFS) is used for feature selection. The goal for choosing features is the maximization of the classification accuracy. We used a weighted classification accuracy due to the uneven class distribution of our data set. This is the rate with which the system is able to correctly identify each class. Then we take an average of these rates with respect to the number of classes. Therefore our overall classification accuracy is defined as:

$$\text{Overall accuracy} = \frac{1}{M} \sum_{j=1}^{M} \frac{\text{correctly\_classified}(C_j)}{\text{number\_of\_test\_images}(C_j)} \tag{3}$$

where M is the number of classes.

A leave-one-out cross-validation method is used during feature selection. Each image is used as a test image, all the remaining images in the training set are ranked according to their similarity index to the test image. Finally the test image is classified to the class which is most frequent among the K samples nearest to it using

Eq. (2). The features that maximize the classification accuracy over all the images in the training set are selected among all the extracted features.

At the end, there will be three sets of features for the three classification tasks, one selected for the top classifier and two selected for the subclassifiers. The feature sets for the two subsystems are also selected using SFS, but only using images from the appropriate classes (i.e. AK/BCC/SCC or ML/SK). Note that, since every subnode in the hierarchy has only a subset of the total classes, and the subnodes each have fewer images, the additional cost of feature selection is not substantially more than that of a flat classification scheme.

3.3 Classification Phase

In the classification phase all the test images are classified through the hierarchical structure. Each image is first classified into one of the two groups by the top level classifier that uses the first set of features. Then one of the classifiers of the second level is invoked according to the output group of the top classifier and therefore the image is classified in one of the 5 diagnostic classes using one of the two other subsets of features.

A drawback of the proposed method is that errors on the first classification level can not be corrected in the second level. If an example is incorrectly classified at the top level and assigned to a group that does not contain the true class, then the classifiers at lower levels have no chance of achieving a correct classification. This is known as the "blocking" problem [58]. An attempt to solve this problem could be to use classifiers on the second level which classify to more than the two or three classes for which they are optimized. Our attempts in this direction show us that not only these classifiers gave much worse results, but also incur additional problems due to the very small number of images wrongly classified in the first level, that makes the classes more unbalanced.

4 Feature Description

Here, skin lesions are characterized by their color and texture. In this section we will describe a set of features that can capture such properties.

4.1 Color Features

Color features are represented by the mean colors $\mu = (\mu_R, \mu_G, \mu_B)$ of the lesion and their covariance matrices Σ. Let

$$\mu_X = \frac{1}{N}\sum_{i=1}^{N} X_i \quad \text{and} \quad C_{XY} = \frac{1}{N}\left[\sum_{i=1}^{N} X_i Y_i\right] - \mu_X \mu_Y \tag{4}$$

where: N is the number of pixels in the lesion, X_i the color component of channel X ($X, Y \in \{R, G, B\}$) of pixel i. In the RGB (Red, Green, Blue) color space, the covariance matrix is:

$$\Sigma = \begin{bmatrix} C_{RR} & C_{RG} & C_{RB} \\ C_{GR} & C_{GG} & C_{GB} \\ C_{BR} & C_{BG} & C_{BB} \end{bmatrix} \tag{5}$$

In this work, RGB, HSV (Hue, Saturation, Value) and CIE_Lab, CIE_Lch (Munsell color coordinate system [48]) and Ohta [46] color spaces were considered. Four normalization techniques were investigated to reduce the impact of lighting, which were applied before extracting color features. In the end, we normalized each color component by dividing each color component by the average of the same component of the healthy skin of the same patient, because it had best performance compared to the other normalization techniques. After experimenting with the 5 different color spaces, we choose the normalized RGB, because it gave slightly better results than the other color spaces (see Sect. 5.4.2)

4.2 Texture Features

Texture features are extracted from generalized co-occurrence matrices (GCM). Assume an image I having N_x columns, N_y rows and N_g gray levels. Let $L_x = \{1, 2, \ldots, N_x\}$ be the columns, $L_y = \{1, 2, \ldots, N_y\}$ be the rows, and $G_x = \{0, 1, \ldots, N_g - 1\}$ be the set of quantized gray levels. The co-occurrence matrix P_δ is a matrix of dimension $N_g \times N_g$, where [30]:

$$P_\delta(i, j) = \#\left\{\left((k, l), (m, n)\right) \in (L_y \times L_x) \times (L_y \times L_x) \mid I(k, l) = i, \ I(m, n) = j\right\} \tag{6}$$

i.e. the number of co-occurrences of the pair of gray levels i and j which are a distance $\delta = (d, \theta)$ apart. In our work, the pixel pairs (k, l) and (m, n) have distance $d = 5, 10, 15, 20, 25, 30$ and orientation $\theta = 0°, 45°, 90°, 135°$, i.e. $(m = k + d, n = l)$, $(m = k + d/\sqrt{2}, n = l + d/\sqrt{2})$, $(m = k, n = l + d)$, $(m = k - d/\sqrt{2}, n = l + d/\sqrt{2})$.

Generalized co-occurrence matrices are the extension of the co-occurrence matrix to multispectral images, i.e. images coded on n color channels [6]. Let u and v be two color channels. The generalized co-occurrence matrices are:

$$P_\delta^{(u,v)}(i, j) = \#\left\{\left((k, l), (m, n)\right) \in (L_y \times L_x) \times (L_y \times L_x) \mid I_u(k, l) = i, \right.$$
$$\left. I_v(m, n) = j\right\} \tag{7}$$

For example, in case of color images, coded on three channels (RGB), we have six cooccurrence matrices: (RR), (GG), (BB) that are the same as gray level co-occurrence matrices computed on one channel and (RG), (RB), (GB) that take into account the correlations between the channels.

Fig. 3 Areas of lesions
where ratio features where
calculated

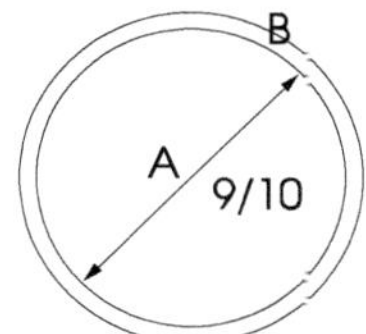

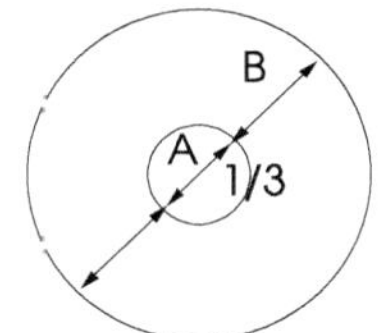

In order to have orientation invariance for our set of GCMs, we averaged the matrices with respect to θ. Quantization levels $N_G = 64, 128, 256$ are used for the three color spaces: *RGB*, *HSV* and *CIE_Lab*.

From each GCM we extracted 12 texture features: energy, contrast, correlation, entropy, homogeneity, inverse difference moment, cluster shade, cluster prominence, max probability, autocorrelation, dissimilarity and variance as defined in [30], for a total of 3888 texture features (12 features $\times$ 6 inter-pixel distances $\times$ 6 color pairs $\times$ 3 color spaces $\times$ 3 gray level quantisations). Two sets of texture features are extracted from GCMs calculated over the lesion area of the image, as well as over a patch of healthy skin of the same image. Differences and ratios of each of the lesion and normal skin values are also calculated, giving 2 more sets of features:

$$feature_{l-s} = feature_{lesion} - feature_{healthy\_skin} \tag{8}$$

$$feature_{l/s} = feature_{lesion} / feature_{healthy\_skin} \tag{9}$$

Altogether, for a given feature family we use $\{feature_{lesion}, feature_{healthy\_skin}, feature_{l-s}, feature_{l/s}\}$. This gives a total of $4 \times 3888 = 15552$ possible texture features, from which we extracted a good subset. All features are z-normalized over all training data.

4.3 Ad Hoc Color Ratio Features

Color ratio features are designed ad hoc for skin lesions, by observing color variations inside the lesion area. Mean colors μ_A and μ_B are extracted over the areas A and B shown in Fig. 3, and their ratios calculated as:

$$ratio = \frac{\mu_A}{\mu_B} \tag{10}$$

Two different area sizes are considered. In the first case, the thickness of the border area is 10 % of the area of the lesion. In the second case, the diameter of the inner area is 1/3 of the diameter of the whole lesion. Since lesions are not circular, the morphological erosion operator is applied iteratively inward from the border until the desired percentages of lesion area pixels are reached. These features seem particularly useful for BCCs, which present pearly edges.

Ad hoc color ratio features are calculated for the three color spaces: *RGB*, *HSV* and *CIE_Lab*, and all feature set are z-normalized. These properties are included in the texture feature set.

4.4 Distance Measure

The color and texture features are combined to construct a distance measure between each test image T and a database image I.

For color covariance-based features, the Bhattacharya distance metric:

$$BD_{CF}(T, I) = \frac{1}{8}(\mu_T - \mu_I)^T \left[\frac{(\Sigma_T + \Sigma_I)}{2}\right]^{-1} (\mu_T - \mu_I) + \frac{1}{2}\ln\frac{|\frac{(\Sigma_T + \Sigma_I)}{2}|}{\sqrt{|\Sigma_T||\Sigma_I|}} \tag{11}$$

is used, where μ_T and μ_I are the average (over all pixels in the lesion) color feature vectors, Σ_T and Σ_I are the covariance matrices of the lesion of T and I respectively, and $|\cdot|$ denotes the matrix determinant.

The Euclidean distance:

$$ED_{TF}(T, I) = \left\| f_{subset}^T - f_{subset}^I \right\| = \sqrt{\sum_{i=1}^{S}(f_i^T - f_i^I)^2} \tag{12}$$

is used for distances between a subset of S texture features f_{subset}, selected as described later. Other metric distances (mahalanobis, cityblock) have been considered, but gave worse results.

We aggregated the two distances into a distance matching function as:

$$Dist(T, I) = w \cdot BD_{CF}(T, I) + (1 - w) \cdot ED_{TF}(T, I) \tag{13}$$

where w is a weighting factor that has been selected experimentally, after trying all the values: $\{0.1, 0.2, \ldots, 0.9\}$. In our case, $w = 0.7$ gave the best results. A low value of $Dist$ indicates a high similarity.

5 Methods

The features described in previous sections were extracted from the lesions in our image database. In this section we will describe in detail the image analysis and the choices of the model parameters.

5.1 Acquisition and Preprocessing

Our image database comprises 960 lesions, belonging to 5 classes (45 AK, 239 BCC, 331 ML, 88 SCC, 257 SK). The ground truth used for the experiments is based on the agreed classifications by 2 dermatologists and a pathologist.

Images are acquired using a Canon EOS 350D SLR camera. Lighting was controlled using a ring flash and all images were captured at the same distance ($\sim$50 cm) resulting in a pixel resolution of about 0.03 mm. Lesions are segmented using the region-based active contour approach described in [39]. The segmentation method uses a statistical model based the level-set framework. Morphological opening has been applied to the segmented lesions to be sure to have patches containing only lesions and healthy skin where the features are extracted.

5.2 Highlight Removal

Specular highlights appear as small and bright regions in various parts of our skin images. The highlights created by specular reflections are a major obstacle for proper color and texture feature extraction.

Specular highlights are often characterized by local coincidence of intense brightness (I) and low color saturation (S). Intensity and saturation are defined as follow:

$$I = \frac{R + G + B}{3} \tag{14}$$

$$S = 1 - \frac{\min(R, G, B)}{I} \tag{15}$$

and candidate specular reflection regions can be identified using appropriate threshold values (motivated by [38]):

$$I > I_{thr} \cdot I_{max} \tag{16}$$

$$S < S_{thr} \cdot S_{max} \tag{17}$$

where I_{max} are S_{max} the maximum intensity and saturation in the image respectively.

The most appropriate threshold values experimentally chosen ($I_{thr} = 0.8$) and ($S_{thr} = 0.5$) differ from the values proposed in [38] probably due to the different nature of the images.

We did not apply any subsequent filling procedure on the detected regions, as this may destroy the original texture and therefore have a negative impact of the subsequent feature extraction. Areas identified as "highlight" were simply excluded from the region where the feature extraction process takes place.

5.3 Feature Normalization

The features described in previous sections have very different value ranges. To account for this, an objective rescaling of the features is achieved by normalizing to z-scores of each feature set, which is defined as

$$z_{ij} = \frac{x_{ij} - \mu_j}{\sigma_j} \tag{18}$$

where: x_{ij} represents the ith sample measure of feature j, μ_j the mean value of all samples for feature j and σ_j is the standard deviation of the samples for feature j.

In addition, feature values outside the values at 5–95 percentiles have been truncated to the 5th or 95th percentile value, and the normalising μ and σ calculated from the truncated set. The normalising parameters were constant over all experiments.

5.4 Evaluation

To assess performance, training and test sets were created by randomly splitting the data set into 3 equal subsets. The only constraint on otherwise random partitioning was that a class was represented equally in each subset. A 3-fold cross-validation method was used, i.e. 3 sets composed of two-thirds of the data were created and used as training sets for feature selection and the remaining one-third of the data as the test set using the selected features for classification. Thus no training example used for feature selection was used as a test example in the same experiment. Three experiments were conducted independently and performance reported as mean and standard deviation over the three experiments.

In the hierarchical classifiers mentioned in previous sections, the most commonly used performance measures are the classic information retrieval notions of precision and recall, or a combination of the two measures [58]. As we are dealing with a classification task and not a retrieval task, we use the classification accuracy derived from the confusion matrix. In the training stage, confusion matrices are obtained by a leave-one-out scheme, where each image is used as a test image and classified according the known classification of the remaining images in the training set. On the other hand, in the classification stage, confusion matrices are obtained in a slightly different way: each image of the test set is classified according to the known classifications of the K nearest neighbors in the training set.

5.4.1 Influence of the K Parameter

Classification results when varying the value of K of the K-NN classifiers have been evaluated. In some experiments we noticed a little improvement by using a smaller value of K for feature selection and a bigger one for classification. Table 1 shows our evaluation. The numbers (mean $\pm$ standard deviation of the accuracy over the three sets) in the first column are obtained in the feature selection stage, *i.e.* using the value of K written on their left. The highest classification accuracy over the test sets for each value of K used during the feature selection are highlighted in boldface.

We chose values of K: (1) to be odd numbers, (2) to be smaller than the training class sizes and (3) to span what seemed like a sensible range. Since performance does not vary too much for the $K = 11$ or $K = 15$ test cases, any value of K in this range is probably approximately equally effective. In the following, the presented

Table 1 Accuracy of the three subclassifiers varying the value of K. Each row shows the value of K used in training, columns show the K used in testing

(a) Top level

	Training Set	Test Set		
		$K = 7$	$K = 11$	$K = 15$
$K = 7$	95.80 ± 0.53	91.67 ± 0.93	**$92\ 09 \pm 1.59$**	91.88 ± 1.23
$K = 11$	95.68 ± 0.18	**93.33 ± 0.67**	$92\ 71 \pm 1.17$	92.61 ± 0.74
$K = 15$	95.73 ± 0.63	93.23 ± 1.42	$93\ 33 \pm 0.95$	**$\underline{93.86 \pm 0.72}$**

(b) Group1 (AK, BCC, SCC)

	Training Set	Test Set		
		$K = 7$	$K = 11$	$K = 15$
$K = 7$	79.40 ± 0.75	69.48 ± 0.98	**$71\ 50 \pm 1.28$**	70.95 ± 2.31
$K = 11$	79.96 ± 3.40	69.07 ± 3.38	$70\ 04 \pm 0.88$	**70.86 ± 1.14**
$K = 15$	81.87 ± 3.62	70.87 ± 0.91	**$\underline{72\ 64 \pm 2.41}$**	71.79 ± 2.06

(c) Group2 (ML, SK)

	Training Set	Test Set		
		$K = 7$	$K = 11$	$K = 15$
$K = 7$	91.97 ± 0.42	85.82 ± 0.88	**$86\ 01 \pm 0.86$**	85.82 ± 0.39
$K = 11$	91.88 ± 0.54	85.64 ± 0.58	$86\ 00 \pm 0.70$	**$\underline{86.19 \pm 0.59}$**
$K = 15$	90.80 ± 1.20	84.55 ± 0.86	**$85\ 84 \pm 0.81$**	85.67 ± 1.43

results are obtained using the combination of K that gave the best classification accuracy (underlined in the table) on the test set for each subclassifier (top level classifier: train $K = 15$, test $K = 15$; AK/BCC/SCC classifier: train $K = 15$, test $K = 11$; ML/SK classifier: train $K = 11$, test $K = 15$). Recalling that K is the number of nearest samples used to classify the image under examination, it is technically correct to use different values at the classification stage than those used during the feature selection stage.

5.4.2 Influence of Color Features

A comparison of the accuracy (mean $\pm$ standard deviation over the three sets) of the three subclassifiers using only color features is reported in Table 2, using the K values reported in the previous section. Note that values for RGB are different from Table 1 because texture features are not used here.

The best results are obtained using RGB and Ohta color spaces. Actually all accuracies are nearly identical before normalization. After normalization, RGB and

Table 2 Accuracy of the three subclassifiers over the three sets using different color spaces, before and after normalization

(a) Before color normalization

	Top level	Group1	Group2
RGB	87.82 ± 2.14	64.37 ± 3.80	55.03 ± 1.31
HSV	87.81 ± 2.21	62.61 ± 2.88	55.03 ± 1.31
Lab	87.20 ± 2.68	63.47 ± 2.73	55.95 ± 1.33
Lch	86.46 ± 2.52	63.48 ± 2.91	55.05 ± 0.62
Ohta	87.82 ± 0.97	64.37 ± 3.80	55.85 ± 1.37

(b) After color normalization

	Top level	Group1	Group2
RGB	92.71 ± 0.66	74.38 ± 1.81	84.35 ± 1.19
HSV	89.80 ± 1.95	62.65 ± 4.16	54.45 ± 2.60
Lab	91.04 ± 1.45	62.93 ± 3.68	56.87 ± 1.94
Lch	87.71 ± 1.80	65.23 ± 3.57	53.54 ± 2.40
Ohta	92.71 ± 0.66	62.31 ± 2.71	57.79 ± 3.40

Ohta color spaces still give best results for the top classifier, while RGB gives much better results for the other two subclassifiers. These data also indicate that color features are more important at the top level of the hierarchy, i.e. in discriminating cancerous vs non cancerous lesions.

5.4.3 Influence of Texture Features

The texture feature set that best discriminates between the groups at the first level of the hierarchy is different from the feature sets that best discriminate at the second level, and these two sets also differ between each other. Figure 4 shows a scatter plot of the two top features for each classifier. The list of selected features for each level of the hierarchy is reported in the Appendix (see Table 8). Considering that a potentially very different set of features is selected at each node of the hierarchy, we can say that the hierarchical method, as a whole, actually uses a larger set of features in a more efficient way, without ending up in problems like the "curse of dimensionality". Hence, there is a benefit from the hierarchical scheme.

We can observe that color information is important also in the texture features because texture properties extracted using different color channels are selected.

The plots of the accuracy vs the number of features (from 1 to 10 for each level of the hierarchy) are shown in Fig. 5. We show only the plots for one of the three subsets and for the best K combinations. Keeping in mind that the color features are fixed and feature selection is applied only to texture features, the nearly flat trend of the top level classifier (Fig. 5 top) confirms that color features are more important in discriminating AK/BCC/SC from ML/SK, and adding more texture features does

Fig. 4 Scatter plots of the top 2 features for each of the three sets. Top graph shows *Group1* (AK/BCC/SCC) in *red* and *Group2* (SK/ML) in *green*

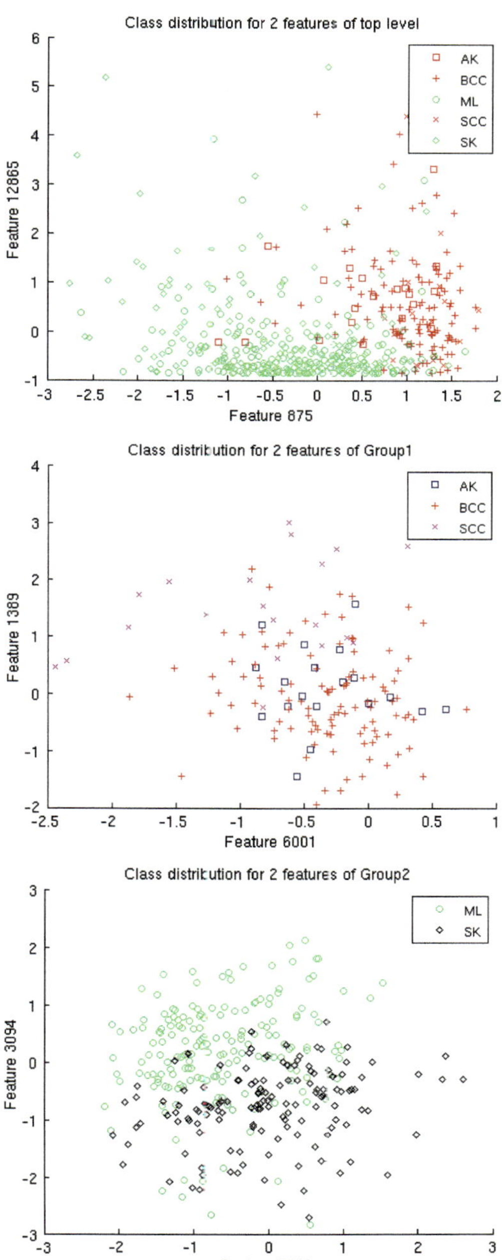

Fig. 5 Plots of accuracy vs number of texture features for one of the 3 subsets, using color feature +1 to 10 texture features

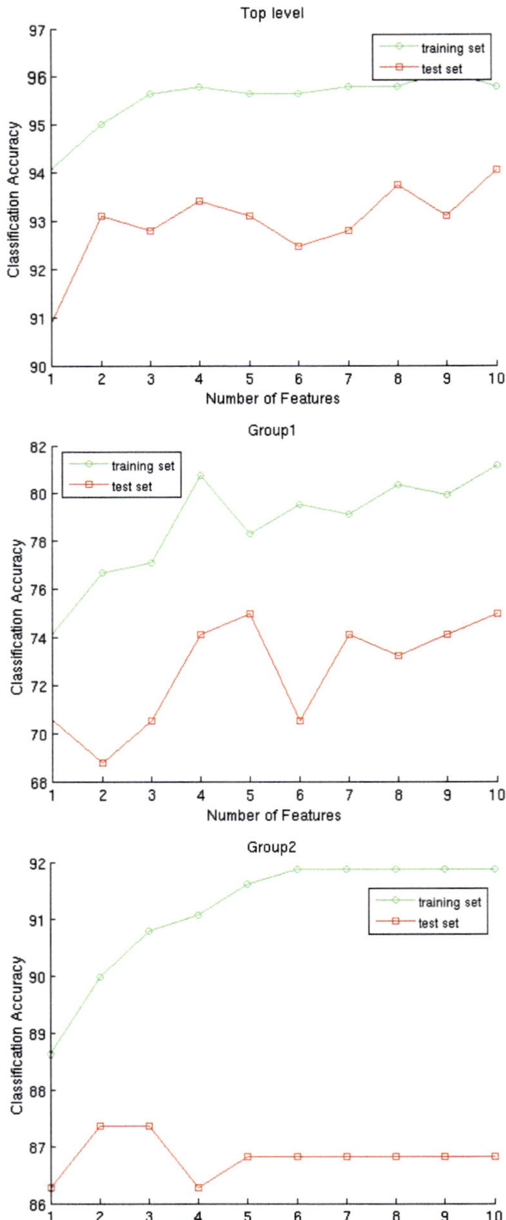

Table 3 Accuracy of the three subclassifiers over the three training sets, validation sets and test sets

(a) Stop when validation accuracy decreases once

	Top level	Group1	Group2
Training set	94.06 ± 1.37	71.63 ± 6.20	87.84 ± 1.01
Validation set	91.88 ± 0.81	69.16 ± 0.36	85.99 ± 0.39
Test set	91.56 ± 1.06	71.49 ± 1.91	86.01 ± 0.33
# Features	5, 5, 3	6, 9, 3	3, 3, 14

(b) Stop when validation accuracy decreases twice

	Top level	Group1	Group2
Training set	94.06 ± 1.90	70.77 ± 6.17	87.56 ± 1.45
Validation set	92.40 ± 0.77	69.69 ± 1.92	86.55 ± 0.70
Test set	90.83 ± 0.94	71.51 ± 2.70	85.32 ± 3.08
# Features	16, 13, 2	5, 18, 2	18, 2, 12

not improve its performance more than 2 %. On the other hand, the trend of the AK/BCC/SCC and ML/SK subclassifiers (Fig. 5 bottom) indicates the usefulness of using texture features at this level of the hierarchy.

5.4.4 Influence of Feature Number and Selection Algorithm

Referring again to the plots shown in Fig. 5, we can see that is reasonable to stop after adding 10 texture features to color features, as the accuracy on the test set was not significantly improving anymore.

A slight overfitting problem evident in some plots suggested us to make experiments using the three sets as train, validation, test sets respectively. Results (mean $\pm$ standard deviation of the accuracy over the three subsets) are reported in Table 3. We stopped selecting additional features when the accuracy on the validation set decreased (once in the top table, twice in the bottom one).

We did not notice any significant improvement. This is probably due to the smaller training set size that further reduced the size of the smallest class.

The number of features selected for each of the three subsets is in the last row of the tables. The high variation means the number of selected features is not a crucial choice. Indeed, the three subsets are created by randomly splitting the data in such a way that the 5 lesion classes were equally represented in each subset.

The SFS feature selection algorithm is claimed not to be the optimal algorithm, however in our case the use of a sequential forward backward greedy algorithm (see Table 4) did not show any significant improvement. Once again we note a high variation in the number of selected features for the three subsets.

Table 4 Accuracy of the three subclassifiers over the three training sets, validation sets and test sets using a greedy forward backward algorithm

	Top level	Group1	Group2
Training set	95.35 ± 1.73	80.25 ± 5.09	91.35 ± 0.40
Validation set	91.67 ± 0.45	67.19 ± 1.67	85.45 ± 0.78
Test set	90.52 ± 0.97	72.08 ± 2.92	86.75 ± 2.55
# Features	5, 20, 10	10, 20, 4	20, 4, 20

Table 5 Comparison of the overall percentage accuracy of the hierarchical and flat classifiers over the three training sets and test sets

	Flat KNN	HKNN	Flat Bayes	Hierarc. Bayes
Training set	77.6 ± 1.4	83.4 ± 1.4	74.3 ± 2.2	81.9 ± 1.5
Test set	69.8 ± 1.6	74.3 ± 2.5	67.7 ± 2.3	69.6 ± 0.4

5.5 Comparison with Other Methods

In Table 5 we compare our results with the results obtained using a non hierarchical approach, i.e. a flat K-NN classifier and a Bayes classifier that use a single set of features for all the 5 classes. The flat classifiers were trained using features selected using the same SFS algorithm. Results of a hierarchical Bayes classifier, having the same hierarchy as the HKNN classifier and whose subclassifiers were trained using the same features and the same SFS algorithm, are also reported in the table. We see that the use of hierarchy gives an improvement both over the training and test sets.

6 Overall Results

The final results are reported in Table 6. The final accuracy of the top classifier and the two subclassifiers at the bottom levels are also reported here. The values are the mean $\pm$ standard deviation over the three training and test sets. These results are obtained using best combination of K determined in Sect. 5.4.1, the RGB color features and 10 texture features for each subclassifier. We decided to use a fixed number of features as the train-validation-test scheme did not enhance performance (see considerations in Sect. 5.4.4 about set sizes and number of features). Similarly, the variety of results from the different configurations and numbers of features all have about the same level, given the estimated standard deviations, and so suggest that there is little risk of overtraining.

Recall the top level classifier discriminates between cancer and pre-malignant conditions (AK/BCC/SCC) and benign forms of skin lesions (ML/SK). Therefore, its very high accuracy (above 93 %) indicates the good performance of our system in identifying cancer and potential at risk conditions. Analysis of the wrongly classified

Table 6 Accuracy of the three subclassifiers and combined classifier over the three training sets and test sets. Note that the Group1/2 results are only over the lesions correctly classified at the top level. On the other hand, the full classifier results report accuracy based on both levels

	Top level	Group1	Group2	Full classifier
Training set	95.7 ± 0.6	81.9 ± 3.6	91.9 ± 0.5	83.4 ± 1.4
Test set	93.9 ± 0.7	72.6 ± 2.4	86.2 ± 0.6	74.3 ± 2.5

Table 7 Classification results: confusion matrix on the test images. Rows are true classes, columns are the selected classes

	AK	BCC	ML	SCC	SK
AK	7	27	1	9	1
BCC	2	210	6	14	7
ML	10	10	269	10	42
SCC	8	34	5	36	5
SK	9	8	33	8	199

images at the top level pointed out that these were the lesions on which clinical diagnosis of experienced dermatologists was most uncertain.

The overall classification accuracy on the test set is 74.3 ± 2.5 %, as shown in the right column of Table 6. The overall result also includes the ~6 % misclassified samples from the first level.

The overall performance (74 %) is not yet at the 90 % level (achieved after 20+ years of research) for differential diagnosis of moles versus melanoma, however, our method addresses lesion classes that seem to have no previous automated image analysis (outside of research from our group [2–4, 8, 9, 36, 39, 65]) and, as highlighted previously, our algorithms' performance is above the diagnostic accuracy currently being achieved by non-specialists.

Table 7 shows the confusion matrix of the whole HKNN system on the test images. This matrix has been obtained by adding the three confusion matrices from the three test sets, as they are disjoint. We note a good percentage of correctly classified BCC, ML and SK. The number of correctly classified AK and SCC at a first glance looks quite low. This is due to the small number of images in each of these two classes. However most of the AKs are misclassified as BCC and we should remember that AK is a pre-malignant lesion. Also many SCC are classified as BCC which is another kind of cancer. Therefore consequences of these mistakes are not as dramatic as if they were diagnosed as benign. An additional split in the hierarchy may improve results.

7 Conclusions

We have presented an algorithm based on a novel hierarchical K-NN classifier, and its application as the first classification of 5 most common classes of non-melanoma skin lesion from color images. Our approach uses a hierarchical combination of three classifiers, utilizing feature selection to tailor the feature set of each classifier to its task. The hierarchical K-NN structure improves the performance of the system over the flat K-NN and a Bayes classifier.

As the accuracy is above 70 %, this system could be used in the future as a diagnostic aid for skin lesion images, particularly as the cancerous vs non cancerous results are ∼94 %.

These results were produced by optimizing classification accuracy. For medical use future research should include the cost of decisions into the optimization process.

Further studies will include the extraction of other texture related features, the evaluation of other feature selection methods and the use of a weighted K-NN model, where neighbor images are weighted according their distance to the test image. In the future, it would be interesting to extend the hierarchical approach to more than two hierarchical levels, including self-learned hierarchies.

Acknowledgement We thank the Wellcome Trust for funding this project (Grant No: 083928/Z/07/Z).

Appendix

List of texture features selected for each level of the final tree. (See Table 8.)

Table 8 Legend: R = Red, G = Green, B = Blue, H = Hue, S = Saturation, V = Value, L, a, b = Lab color space. Texture features are defined in [30]

(a) Top level

Texture feature	Interp. distance	Quant. levels	Color channels	Site
Entropy	5	128	HV	Lesion
Cluster Shade	10	128	Lb	Skin
Inv. Diff. Moment	5	64	SV	Lesion
Contrast	15	64	ab	Skin
Energy	5	64	HV	Lesion
Inv. Diff. Moment	15	64	RG	Lesion
Max Probability	5	128	HH	Lesion/skin
Cluster Prominence	25	64	GG	Skin
Correlation	10	256	HV	Lesion
Cluster Prominence	15	64	LL	Lesion-skin

Table 8 (Continued)

(b) Group 1 (AK,BCC,SCC)

Texture feature	Interp. distance	Quant. levels	Color channels	Site
Variance	30	64	HS	Lesion/skin
Energy	25	256	ab	Lesion
Inv. Diff. Moment	25	64	BB	Lesion
Entropy	15	128	HH	Lesion
Max Probability	5	256	RB	Lesion/skin
Cluster Prominence	10	64	SS	Lesion-skin
Contrast	5	64	SS	Lesion
Homogeneity	15	256	RG	Lesion
Homogeneity	25	128	SV	Lesion/skin
Inv. Diff. Moment	5	64	HS	Skin

(c) Group 2 (ML,SK)

Texture feature	Interp. distance	Quant. levels	Color channels	Site
Correlation	10	256	SS	Lesion
Dissimilarity	5	64	bb	Skin
Cluster Shade	5	64	HH	Lesion
Cluster Shade	5	64	HV	Lesion
Cluster Prominence	5	64	HH	Lesion
Cluster Prominence	5	64	HS	Lesion
Cluster Shade	10	64	HV	Lesion
Cluster Shade	5	256	HV	Lesion
Correlation	5	64	HV	Skin
Contrast	5	64	HH	Lesion

References

1. Alcón JF, Heinrich A, Uzunbajakava N, Krekels G, Siem D, de Haan G, de Haan G (2009) Automatic imaging system with decision support for inspection of pigmented skin lesions and melanoma diagnosis. IEEE J Sel Top Signal Process 3:14–25
2. Aldridge RB, Glodzik D, Ballerini L, Fisher RB, Rees JL (2011) The utility of non-rule-based visual matching as a strategy to allow novices to achieve skin lesion diagnosis. Acta Derm-Venereol 91:279–283
3. Aldridge RB, Li X, Ballerini L, Fisher RB, Rees JL (2010) Teaching dermatology using 3-dimensional virtual reality. Archives of Dermatology 149(10)
4. Aldridge RB, Zanotto M, Ballerini L, Fisher RB, Rees JL (2011) Novice identification of melanoma: not quite as straightforward as the ABCDs. Acta Derm-Venereol 91:125–130
5. Armengol E (2011) Classification of melanomas in situ using knowledge discovery with explained case-based reasoning. Artif Intell Med 51:93–105
6. Arvis V, Debain C, Berducat M, Benassi A (2004) Generalization of the cooccurence matrix for colour images: application to colour texture classification. Image Anal Stereol 23(1):63–72

7. Aslandogan Y, Mahajani G (2004) Evidence combination in medical data mining. In: Proceedings of international conference on information technology: coding and computing, vol 2, pp 465–469

8. Ballerini L, Li X, Fisher RB, Aldridge B, Rees J (2010) Content-based image retrieval of skin lesions by evolutionary feature synthesis. In: di Chio C, et al (eds) Application of evolutionary computation, Istanbul, Turkey. Lectures notes in computer science, vol 6024, pp 312–319

9. Ballerini L, Li X, Fisher RB, Rees J (2010) A query-by-example content-based image retrieval system of non-melanoma skin lesions. In: Caputo B (ed) Proceedings MICCAI-09 workshop MCBR-CDS 2009: medical content-based retrieval for clinical decision support. LNCS, vol 5853. Springer, Berlin, pp 31–38

10. Basarab T, Munn S, Jones RR (1996) Diagnostic accuracy and appropriateness of general practitioner referrals to a dermatology out-patient clinic. Br J Dermatol 135(1):70–73

11. Cascinelli N, Ferrario M, Tonelli T, Leo E (1987) A possible new tool for clinical diagnosis of melanoma: the computer. J Am Acad Dermatol 16(2):361–367

12. Cavalcanti PG, Scharcanski J (2011) Automated prescreening of pigmented skin lesions using standard cameras. Comput Med Imaging Graph 35(6):481–491

13. Ceci M, Malerba D (2003) Hierarchical classification of HTML documents with WebClassII. In: Proceedings of the 25th European conference on information retrieval, pp 57–72

14. Celebi ME, Iyatomi H, Schaefer G, Stoecker WV (2009) Lesion border detection in dermoscopy images. Comput Med Imaging Graph 33(2):148–153

15. Celebi ME, Kingravi HA, Uddin B, Iyatomi H, Aslandogan YA, Stoecker WV, Moss RH (2007) A methodological approach to the classification of dermoscopy images. Comput Med Imaging Graph 31(6):362–373

16. Celebi ME, Stoecker WV, Moss RH (2011) Advances in skin cancer image analysis. Comput Med Imaging Graph 35(2):83–84

17. Cover T, Hart P (1967) Nearest neighbor pattern classification. IEEE Trans Inf Theory 13(1):21–27

18. Cancer research UK (CRUK). CancerStats, Internet (2011). URL http://info.cancerresearchuk.org/cancerstats. Accessed 03/08/2011

19. Dalal A, Moss RH, Stanley RJ, Stoecker WV, Gupta K, Calcara DA, Xu J, Shrestha B, Drugge R, Malters JM, Perry LA (2011) Concentric decile segmentation of white and hypopigmented areas in dermoscopy images of skin lesions allows discrimination of malignant melanoma. Comput Med Imaging Graph 35(2):148–154

20. D'Alessio S, Murray K, Schiaffino R, Kershenbaum A (2000) The effect of using hierarchical classifiers in text categorization. In: Proceedings of 6th international conference recherche d'information assistee par ordinateur, pp 302–313

21. Day GR, Barbour RH (2000) Automated melanoma diagnosis: where are we at? Skin Res Technol 6:1–5

22. Dimitrovski I, Kocev D, Loskovska S, Dzeroski S (2011) Hierarchical annotation of medical images. Pattern Recognit 44(10–11):2436–2449

23. Dumais S, Chen H (2000) Hierarchical classification of web content. In: Proceedings of the 23rd annual international ACM SIGIR conference on research and development in information retrieval. ACM, New York, pp 256–263

24. Duwairi R, Al-Zubaidi R (2011) A hierarchical K-NN classifier for textual data. Int Arab J Inf Technol 8(3):251–259

25. Fix E, Hodges JL (1989) Discriminatory analysis. Nonparametric discrimination: consistency properties. Int Stat Rev 57(3):238–247

26. Garnavi R, Aldeen M, Celebi ME, Varigos G, Finch S (2011) Border detection in dermoscopy images using hybrid thresholding on optimized color channels. Comput Med Imaging Graph 35(2):105–115

27. Gerbert B, Maurer T, Berger T, Pantilat S, McPhee SJ, Wolff M, Bronstone A, Caspers N (1996) Primary care physicians as gatekeepers in managed care: primary care physicians' and dermatologists' skills at secondary prevention of skin cancer. Arch Dermatol 132(9):1030–1038

28. Gordon AD (1987) A review of hierarchical classification. J R Stat Soc A 150(2):119–137
29. Green A, Martin N, McKenzie G, Pfitzner J, Quintarelli F, Thomas BW, O'Rourke M, Knight N (1991) Computer image analysis of pigmented skin lesions. Melanoma Res 1:231–236
30. Haralick RM, Shanmungam K, Dinstein I (1973) Textural features for image classification. IEEE Trans Syst Man Cybern 3(6):610–621
31. Hintz-madsen M, Hansen LK, Larsen J, Olesen E, Drzewiecki KT (1995) Design and evaluation of neural classifiers application to skin lesion classificat on. In: Proceedings of the 1995 IEEE workshop on neural networks for signal processing V, pp 484–493
32. Iyatomi H, Celebi ME, Schaefer G, Tanaka M (2011) Automated color calibration method for dermoscopy images. Comput Med Imaging Graph 35(2):89–98
33. Jain AK, Duin RPW, Mao J (2000) Statistical pattern recognition: a review. IEEE Trans Pattern Anal Mach Intell 22(1):4–37
34. Jain AK, Zongker D (1997) Feature-selection: evaluation, application, and small sample performance. IEEE Trans Pattern Anal Mach Intell 19(2):153–158
35. Ko CB, Walton S, Keczkes K, Bury HPR, Nicholson C (1994) The emerging epidemic of skin cancer. Br J Dermatol 130:269–272
36. Laskaris N, Ballerini L, Fisher RB, Aldridge B, Rees J (2010) Fuzzy description of skin lesions. In: Manning DJ, Abbey CK (eds) Medical imaging 2010: image perception, observer performance, and technology assessment. Proceedings of the SPIE, vol 7627, pp 762,717-1–762,717-10
37. Lee TK, Claridge E (2005) Predictive power of irregular border shapes for malignant melanomas. Skin Res Technol 11(1):1–8
38. Lehmann TM, Palm C (2001) Color line search for illuminant estimation in real-world scenes. J Opt Soc Am A 18(11):2679–2691
39. Li X, Aldridge B, Ballerini L, Fisher R, Rees J (2009) Depth data improves skin lesion segmentation. In: Proceedings of the 12th international conference on medical image computing and computer assisted intervention (MICCAI), London, pp 1100–1107
40. Maglogiannis I, Doukas CN (2009) Overview of advanced computer vision systems for skin lesions characterization. IEEE Trans Inf Technol Biomed 13(5):721–733
41. Maglogiannis I, Pavlopoulos S, Koutsouris D (2005) An integrated computer supported acquisition, handling, and characterization system for pigmented skin lesions in dermatological images. IEEE Trans Inf Technol Biomed 9(1):86–98
42. Martínez-Otzeta JM, Sierra B, Lazkano E, Astigarraga A (2006) Classifier hierarchy learning by means of genetic algorithms. Pattern Recognit Lett 27(16):1998–2004
43. Mete M, Kockara S, Aydin K (2011) Fast density-based lesion detection in dermoscopy images. Comput Med Imaging Graph 35(2):128–136
44. Morrison A, O'Loughlin S, Powell FC (2001) Suspected skin malignancy: a comparison of diagnoses of family practitioners and dermatologists in 493 patients. Int J Dermatol 40(2):104–107
45. Murtagh F (1983) A survey of recent advances in hierarchical clustering algorithms. Comput J 26(4):354–359
46. Ohta YI, Kanade T, Sakai T (1980) Color information for region segmentation. Comput Graph Image Process 13(1):222–241
47. Pourghassem H, Ghassemian H (2008) Content-based medical image classification using a new hierarchical merging scheme. Comput Med Imaging Graph 32(8):651–661
48. Rahman MM, Desai BC, Bhattacharya P (2006) Image retrieval-based decision support system for dermatoscopic images. In: IEEE symposium on computer-based medical systems. IEEE Computer Society, Los Alamitos, pp 285–290
49. Rigel DS, Russak J, Friedman R (2010) The evolution of melanoma diagnosis: 25 years beyond the ABCDs. CA: Cancer J Clinicians 60(5):301–316
50. Rodriguez C, Boto F, Soraluze I, Pérez A (2002) An incremental and hierarchical K-NN classifier for handwritten characters. In: Proceedings of the 16th international conference on pattern recognition (ICPR'02), vol 3. IEEE Computer Society, Washington, pp 98–101

51. Rosado B, Menzies S, Harbauer A, Pehamberger H, Wolff K, Binder M, Kittler H (2003) Accuracy of computer diagnosis of melanoma: a quantitative meta-analysis. Arch Dermatol 139(3):361–367
52. Sadeghi M, Razmara M, Lee TK, Atkins M (2011) A novel method for detection of pigment network in dermoscopic images using graphs. Comput Med Imaging Graph 35(2):137–143
53. Salah B, Alshraideh M, Beidas R, Hayajneh F (2011) Skin cancer recognition by using a neuro-fuzzy system. Cancer Inform 10:1–11
54. Schaefer G, Rajab MI, Celebi ME, Iyatomi H (2011) Colour and contrast enhancement for improved skin lesion segmentation. Comput Med Imaging Graph 35(2):99–104
55. Schmid-Saugeons P, Guillod J, Thiran JP (2003) Towards a computer-aided diagnosis system for pigmented skin lesions. Comput Med Imaging Graph 27:65–78
56. Seidenari S, Pellacani G, Pepe P (1998) Digital videomicroscopy improves diagnostic accuracy for melanoma. J Am Acad Dermatol 39(2):175–181
57. Stoecker WV, Wronkiewiecz M, Chowdhury R, Stanley RJ, Xu J, Bangert A, Shrestha B, Calcara DA, Rabinovitz HS, Oliviero M, Ahmed F, Perry LA, Drugge R (2011) Detection of granularity in dermoscopy images of malignant melanoma using color and texture features. Comput Med Imaging Graph 35(2):144–147
58. Sun A, Lim EP, Ng WK (2003) Performance measurement framework for hierarchical text classification. J Am Soc Inf Sci Technol 54:1014–1028
59. Tommasi T, Dedelaers T (2010) In: The medical image classification task. ImageCLEF: the information retrieval series, vol 32, pp 221–238
60. Viola KV, Tolpinrud WL, Gross CP, Kirsner RS, Imaeda S, Federman DG (2011) Outcomes of referral to dermatology for suspicious lesions: implications for teledermatology. Arch Dermatol 147(5):556–560
61. Wang H, Moss RH, Chen X, Stanley RJ, Stoecker WV, Celebi ME, Malters JM, Grichnik JM, Marghoob AA, Rabinovitz HS, Menzies SW, Szalapski TM (2011) Modified watershed technique and post-processing for segmentation of skin lesions in dermoscopy images. Comput Med Imaging Graph 35(2):116–120
62. Wettschereck D, Aha DW, Mohri T (1997) A review and empirical evaluation of feature weighting methods for a class of lazy learning algorithms. Artif Intell Rev 11:273–314
63. Wollina U, Burroni M, Torricelli R, Gilardi S, Dell'Eva G, Helm C, Bardey W (2007) Digital dermoscopy in clinical practise: a three-centre analysis. Skin Res Technol 13:133–142
64. Zanotto M (2010) Visual description of skin lesions. Master's thesis, School of Informatics, University of Edinburgh
65. Zanotto M, Ballerini L, Aldridge B, Fisher RB, Rees J (2011) Visual cues do not improve skin lesion ABC(D) grading. In: Manning DJ, Abbey CK (eds) Medical imaging 2011: image perception, observer performance, and technology assessment. Proceedings of the SPIE, vol 7966, pp 79,660U-1–79,660U-10
66. Zhou H, Schaefer G, Celebi ME, Lin F, Liu T (2011) Gradient vector flow with mean shift for skin lesion segmentation. Comput Med Imaging Graph 35(2):121–127

Color Quantization of Dermoscopy Images Using the K-Means Clustering Algorithm

M. Emre Celebi, Quan Wen, Sae Hwang, and Gerald Schaefer

Abstract Color quantization (CQ) is an important operation with various applications in medical image analysis. Most quantization methods are essentially based on data clustering algorithms. However, despite its popularity as a general purpose clustering algorithm, k-means has not received much respect in the CQ literature because of its high computational requirements and sensitivity to initialization. In this chapter, we investigate the performance of a recently proposed k-means based CQ method. Experiments on a diverse set of dermoscopy images of skin lesions demonstrate that an efficient implementation of k-means with an appropriate initialization strategy can in fact serve as a very effective color quantizer.

1 Introduction

True-color images typically contain thousands of colors, which makes their display, storage, transmission, and processing problematic. For this reason, CQ is commonly used as a preprocessing step for various graphics and image processing tasks. In the past, CQ was a necessity due to the limitations of the display hardware, which could not handle over 16 million possible colors in 24-bit images. Although 24-bit display hardware has become more common, CQ still maintains its practical value [8].

M.E. Celebi (✉)
Department of Computer Science, Louisiana State University, Shreveport, LA, USA
e-mail: ecelebi@lsus.edu

Q. Wen
School of Computer Science and Engineering, University of Electronic Science and Technology
of China, Chengdu, P.R. China
e-mail: quanwen@uestc.edu.cn

S. Hwang
Department of Computer Science, University of Illinois, Springfield, IL, USA
e-mail: shwan2@uis.edu

G. Schaefer
Department of Computer Science, Loughborough University, Loughborough, UK
e-mail: gerald.schaefer@ieee.org

M.E. Celebi, G. Schaefer (eds.), *Color Medical Image Analysis*,
Lecture Notes in Computational Vision and Biomechanics 6,
DOI 10.1007/978-94-007-5389-1_5, © Springer Science+Business Media Dordrecht 2013

Modern applications of CQ in graphics and image processing include: (i) compression [74], (ii) segmentation [18], (iii) text localization/detection [60], (iv) color-texture analysis [59], (v) watermarking [42], (vi) non-photorealistic rendering [66], and (vii) content-based retrieval [19].

The process of CQ is mainly comprised of two phases: palette design (the selection of a small set of colors that represents the original image colors) and pixel mapping (the assignment of each input pixel to one of the palette colors). The primary objective is to reduce the number of unique colors, N', in an image to K ($K \ll N'$) with minimal distortion. In most applications, 24-bit pixels in the original image are reduced to 8 bits or fewer. Since natural images often contain a large number of colors, faithful representation of these images with a limited size palette is a difficult problem.

CQ methods can be broadly classified into two categories [71]: image-independent methods that determine a universal (fixed) palette without regard to any specific image [26, 48], and image-dependent methods that determine a custom (adaptive) palette based on the color distribution of the images. Despite being very fast, image-independent methods usually give poor results since they do not take into account the image contents. Therefore, most of the studies in the literature consider only image-dependent methods, which strive to achieve a better balance between computational efficiency and visual quality of the quantization output.

Numerous image-dependent CQ methods have been developed over the past three decades. These can be categorized into two families: preclustering methods and postclustering methods [8]. Preclustering methods are mostly based on the statistical analysis of the color distribution of the images. Divisive preclustering methods start with a single cluster that contains all N' image colors. This initial cluster is recursively subdivided until K clusters are obtained. Well-known divisive methods include median-cut [30], octree [27], variance-based method [65], binary splitting [49], greedy orthogonal bipartitioning [68], optimal principal multilevel quantizer [69], center-cut [37], and rwm-cut [75]. More recent methods can be found in [15, 31, 38, 46, 61]. On the other hand, agglomerative preclustering methods [3, 7, 21, 24, 63, 72] start with N' singleton clusters each of which contains one image color. These clusters are repeatedly merged until K clusters remain. In contrast to preclustering methods that compute the palette only once, postclustering methods first determine an initial palette and then improve it iteratively. Essentially, any data clustering method can be used for this purpose. Since these methods involve iterative or stochastic optimization, they can obtain higher quality results when compared to preclustering methods at the expense of increased computational time. Clustering algorithms adapted to CQ include maxmin [28, 70], k-means [11, 32, 33, 35, 40], k-harmonic means [23], competitive learning [10, 13, 57, 64], fuzzy c-means [9, 41, 50, 55, 67], rough c-means [54, 56], BIRCH [5], and self-organizing maps [14, 16, 17, 51, 53, 73].

In this chapter, we investigate the applicability of a recently proposed k-means based CQ method to dermoscopy image quantization. The rest of the chapter is organized as follows. Section 2 describes the conventional k-means algorithm and the proposed modifications. Section 3 describes the experimental setup and compares the modified k-means CQ method to other methods. Finally, Sect. 4 gives the conclusions and future work.

2 Color Quantization Using K-Means Clustering Algorithm

2.1 K-Means Clustering Algorithm

K-means (KM) is undoubtedly the most widely used partitional clustering algorithm [25]. Given a data set $\mathcal{X} = \{\mathbf{x}_1, \mathbf{x}_2, \ldots, \mathbf{x}_N\} \in \mathbb{R}^D$, the objective of KM is to partition $\mathcal{X}$ into K exhaustive and mutually exclusive clusters $\mathcal{S} = \{S_1, S_2, \ldots, S_K\} \bigcup_{k=1}^{K} S_k = \mathcal{X}$, $S_i \cap S_j = \emptyset$ for $1 \leq i \neq j \leq K$ by minimizing the Sum of Squared Error (SSE):

$$\text{SSE} = \sum_{k=1}^{K} \sum_{\mathbf{x}_i \in S_k} \|\mathbf{x}_i - \mathbf{c}_k\|_2^2 \tag{1}$$

where $\|.\|_2$ denotes the Euclidean ($\mathcal{L}_2$) norm and $\mathbf{c}_k$ is the center of cluster S_k calculated as the mean of the points that belong to this cluster. This problem is known to be NP-hard even for $K = 2$ [1] or $D = 2$ [47], but a heuristic method developed by Lloyd [45] offers a simple solution. Lloyd's algorithm starts with K arbitrary centers, typically chosen uniformly at random from the data points. Each point is then assigned to the nearest center, and each center is recalculated as the mean of all points assigned to it. These two steps are repeated until a predefined termination criterion is met. The pseudocode for this procedure is given in Algorithm 1 (**bold** symbols denote vectors). Here, $m[i]$ denotes the membership of point $\mathbf{x}_i$, i.e., index of the cluster center that is nearest to $\mathbf{x}_i$.

The complexity of KM is $\mathcal{O}(NK)$ per iteration for a fixed D value. In CQ applications D typically equals three since the clustering procedure is often performed in three-dimensional color spaces such as RGB or CIELAB [12].

From a clustering perspective KM has the following advantages:

- It is conceptually simple, versatile, and easy to implement.
- It has a time/space complexity that is linear in N and K. Furthermore, numerous acceleration techniques are available in the literature [20, 29, 36, 39, 43, 52].
- It is guaranteed to terminate [58] and its convergence rate is quadratic [6].
- It is invariant to data ordering, i.e., random shufflings of the data points.

The main disadvantages of KM are the facts that it often terminates at a local minimum [58] and that its output is sensitive to the initial choice of the cluster centers. From a CQ perspective, KM has two additional drawbacks. First, despite its linear time complexity, the iterative nature of the algorithm renders the palette generation phase computationally expensive. Second, the pixel mapping phase is inefficient, since for each input pixel a full search of the palette is required to determine the nearest color. In contrast, preclustering methods often manipulate and store the

input : $\mathcal{X} = \{\mathbf{x}_1, \mathbf{x}_2, \ldots, \mathbf{x}_N\} \in \mathbb{R}^D$ ($N \times D$ input data set)
output: $\mathcal{C} = \{\mathbf{c}_1, \mathbf{c}_2, \ldots, \mathbf{c}_K\} \in \mathbb{R}^D$ (K cluster centers)
Select a random subset $\mathcal{C}$ of $\mathcal{X}$ as the initial set of cluster centers;
while *termination criterion is not met* **do**
    for $(i = 1; i \leq N; i = i + 1)$ **do**
        `Assign` $\mathbf{x}_i$ `to the nearest cluster;`
        $m[i] = \underset{k \in \{1,2,\ldots,K\}}{\text{argmin}} \ \|\mathbf{x}_i - \mathbf{c}_k\|^2;$
    end
    `Recalculate the cluster centers;`
    for $(k = 1; k \leq K; k = k + 1)$ **do**
        `Cluster` S_k `contains the set of points` $\mathbf{x}_i$ `that are`
        `nearest to the center` $\mathbf{c}_k$`;`
        $S_k = \{\mathbf{x}_i \mid m[i] = k\};$
        `Calculate the new center` $\mathbf{c}_k$ `as the mean of the points`
        `that belong to` S_k`;`
        $\mathbf{c}_k = \frac{1}{|S_k|} \sum_{\mathbf{x}_i \in S_k} \mathbf{x}_i;$
    end
end

Algorithm 1: Conventional K-means algorithm

palette in a special data structure (binary trees are commonly used), which allows for fast nearest neighbor search during the mapping phase. Note that these drawbacks are shared by the majority of postclustering methods and will be addressed in the following subsection.

2.2 Modifications to the K-Means Algorithm

We have recently proposed a fast and exact KM variant called *Weighted Sort-Means (WSM)* that is more suitable for CQ [11]. In order to keep the manuscript self-contained, here we present a brief overview of WSM. WSM differs from the conventional KM algorithm as follows:

1. **Data sampling**: A straightforward way to speed up KM is to reduce the amount of data, which can be achieved by subsampling the input image data. In this study, two deterministic subsampling methods are utilized. The first method involves a 2:1 subsampling in the horizontal and vertical directions, so that only 1/4-th of the input image pixels are taken into account [28]. This kind of moderate sampling has been found to be effective in reducing the computational time without degrading the quality of quantization [4, 22, 28, 38]. The second method involves sampling only the pixels with unique colors. These pixels can be determined efficiently using a hash table that uses chaining for collision resolution and a universal hash function of the form: $h_{\mathbf{a}}(\mathbf{x}) = (\sum_{i=1}^{3} a_i x_i) \bmod m$, where $\mathbf{x} = (x_1, x_2, x_3)$ denotes a pixel with red (x_1), green (x_2), and blue (x_3) components, m is a prime number, and the elements of sequence $\mathbf{a} = (a_1, a_2, a_3)$

are chosen randomly from the set $\{0, 1, \ldots, m - 1\}$. This second subsampling method further reduces the image data since most images contain a large number of duplicate colors.

2. **Sample weighting**: An important disadvantage of the second subsampling method described above is that it disregards the color distribution of the original image. In order to address this problem, each point is assigned a weight that is proportional to its frequency. Note that this weighting procedure essentially generates a one-dimensional color histogram. The weights are then normalized by the number of pixels in the image to avoid numerical instabilities in the calculations. In addition, Algorithm 1 is modified to incorporate the weights in the clustering procedure.

3. **Sort-Means algorithm**: The assignment phase of KM involves many redundant distance calculations. In particular, for each point, the distances to each of the K cluster centers are calculated. Consider a point $\mathbf{x}_i$, two cluster centers $\mathbf{c}_a$ and $\mathbf{c}_b$ and a distance metric $d(\cdot, \cdot)$, using the triangle inequality, we have $d(\mathbf{c}_a, \mathbf{c}_b) \leq d(\mathbf{x}_i, \mathbf{c}_a) + d(\mathbf{x}_i, \mathbf{c}_b)$. Therefore, if we know that $2d(\mathbf{x}_i, \mathbf{c}_a) \leq d(\mathbf{c}_a, \mathbf{c}_b)$, we can conclude that $d(\mathbf{x}_i, \mathbf{c}_a) \leq d(\mathbf{x}_i, \mathbf{c}_b)$ without having to calculate $d(\mathbf{x}_i, \mathbf{c}_b)$. The compare-means algorithm [52] precalculates the pairwise distances between cluster centers at the beginning of each iteration. When searching for the nearest cluster center for each point, the algorithm often avoids a large number of distance calculations with the help of the triangle inequality test. The sort-means (SM) algorithm [52] further reduces the number of distance calculations by sorting the distance values associated with each cluster center in ascending order. In each iteration, point $\mathbf{x}_i$ is compared against the cluster centers in increasing order of distance from the center $\mathbf{c}_k$ that $\mathbf{x}_i$ was assigned to in the previous iteration. If a center that is far enough from $\mathbf{c}_k$ is reached, all of the remaining centers can be skipped and the procedure continues with the next point. In this way, SM avoids the overhead of going through all of the centers. It should be noted that more elaborate approaches to accelerate KM have been proposed in the literature. These include algorithms based on kd-trees [39, 43], and more sophisticated uses of the triangle inequality [20, 29]. Some of these algorithms [20, 29] are not suitable for low dimensional data sets such as color image data since they incur significant overhead to create and update auxiliary data structures [20]. Others [39, 43] provide computational gains comparable to SM at the expense of significant conceptual and implementation complexity. In contrast, SM is conceptually simple, easy to implement, and incurs very small overhead, which makes it an ideal candidate for color clustering.

4. **Initialization**: It is well-known that KM is quite sensitive to initialization. Adverse effects of improper initialization include [11]: (i) empty clusters (a.k.a. 'dead units'), (ii) slower convergence, and (iii) a higher chance of getting stuck in bad local minima. Conventional KM algorithm is often initialized by K cluster centers chosen uniformly at random from the data points. Such a random initialization method not only exhibits the aforementioned problems, but also leads to clusterings with highly variable quality. In this study,

the greedy orthogonal bipartitioning method of Wu [68] is used to initialize the cluster centers. This deterministic method has been shown to be one of the most effective and efficient preclustering methods in various studies [10, 11, 13].

The pseudocode for WSM is given in Algorithm 2. Let γ be the average over all points p of the number of centers that are no more than two times as far as p is from the center p was assigned to in the previous iteration. The complexity of WSM is $\mathcal{O}(K^2 + K^2 \log K + N'\gamma)$ per iteration for a fixed D value, where the terms (from left to right) represent the cost of calculating the pairwise distances between the cluster centers, the cost of sorting the centers, and the cost of comparisons, respectively. Here, the last term dominates the computational time, since in CQ applications K is a small number and furthermore $K \ll N'$. Therefore, it can be concluded that WSM is linear in N', the number of unique colors in the original image. It should be noted that, when initialized with the same centers, WSM gives identical results to KM.

3 Experimental Results and Discussion

3.1 Image Set and Performance Criteria

The WSM method was tested on a set of eight true-color (24-bit) dermoscopy images of skin lesions obtained from the EDRA Interactive Atlas of Dermoscopy [2]. The images are shown in Fig. 1.

The effectiveness of a quantization method was quantified by the commonly used Mean Absolute Error (MAE) and Mean Squared Error (MSE) measures:

$$\mathrm{MAE}(\mathbf{X}, \hat{\mathbf{X}}) = \frac{1}{HW} \sum_{h=1}^{H} \sum_{w=1}^{W} \left\| \mathbf{X}(h, w) - \hat{\mathbf{X}}(h, w) \right\|_1$$

$$\mathrm{MSE}(\mathbf{X}, \hat{\mathbf{X}}) = \frac{1}{HW} \sum_{h=1}^{H} \sum_{w=1}^{W} \left\| \mathbf{X}(h, w) - \hat{\mathbf{X}}(h, w) \right\|_2^2 \tag{2}$$

where $\mathbf{X}$ and $\hat{\mathbf{X}}$ denote respectively the $H \times W$ original and quantized images in the RGB color space. MAE and MSE represent the average color distortion with respect to the $\mathcal{L}_1$ (City-block) and $\mathcal{L}_2^2$ (squared Euclidean) norms, respectively. Note that most of the other popular evaluation measures used in the CQ literature such as Peak Signal-to-Noise Ratio (PSNR), Normalized MSE, Root MSE, and average color distortion [51, 64] are variants of either MAE or MSE.

The efficiency of a quantization method was measured by CPU time in milliseconds, which includes the time required for both the palette generation and pixel mapping phases. In order to perform a fair comparison, the fast pixel mapping algorithm described in [34] was used in quantization methods that lack an efficient pixel

input : $\mathcal{X} = \{\mathbf{x}_1, \mathbf{x}_2, \ldots, \mathbf{x}_{N'}\} \in \mathbb{R}^D$ ($N' \times D$ input data set)
$\qquad \mathcal{W} = \{w_1, w_2, \ldots, w_{N'}\} \in [0, 1]$ (N' point weights)
output: $\mathcal{C} = \{\mathbf{c}_1, \mathbf{c}_2, \ldots, \mathbf{c}_K\} \in \mathbb{R}^D$ (K cluster centers)
Select a random subset $\mathcal{C}$ of $\mathcal{X}$ as the initial set of cluster centers;
while *termination criterion is not met* **do**

    Calculate the pairwise distances between the cluster centers;
    for $(i = 1; i \leq K; i = i + 1)$ **do**
        for $(j = i + 1; j \leq K; j = j + 1)$ **do**
            $d[i][j] = d[j][i] = \|\mathbf{c}_i - \mathbf{c}_j\|^2$;
        end
    end
    Construct a $K \times K$ matrix M in which row i is a permutation of $1, 2, \ldots, K$ that represents the clusters in increasing order of distance of their centers from $\mathbf{c}_i$;
    for $(i = 1; i \leq N'; i = i + 1)$ **do**
        Let S_p be the cluster that $\mathbf{x}_i$ was assigned to in the previous iteration;
        $p = m[i]$;
        min_dist $= prev\_dist = \|\mathbf{x}_i - \mathbf{c}_p\|^2$;
        Update the nearest center if necessary;
        for $(j = 2; j \leq K; j = j + 1)$ **do**
            $t = M[p][j]$;
            if $d[p][t] \geq 4\, prev\_dist$ **then**
                There can be no other closer center. Stop checking;
                break;
            end
            dist $= \|\mathbf{x}_i - \mathbf{c}_t\|^2$;
            if $dist \leq min\_dist$ **then**
                $\mathbf{c}_t$ is closer to $\mathbf{x}_i$ than $\mathbf{c}_p$;
                min_dist $=$ dist;
                $m[i] = t$;
            end
        end
    end
    Recalculate the cluster centers;
    for $(k = 1; k \leq K; k = k + 1)$ **do**
        Calculate the new center $\mathbf{c}_k$ as the weighted mean of points that are nearest to it;
        $\mathbf{c}_k = \left(\sum\limits_{m[i]=k} w_i \mathbf{x}_i \right) \Big/ \sum\limits_{m[i]=k} w_i$;
    end
end

Algorithm 2: Weighted sort-means algorithm

mapping phase. All of the programs were implemented in the C language, compiled with the `gcc` v4.4.5 compiler, and executed on an Intel Core i7-980X 3.33 GHz machine. The time figures were averaged over 100 runs.

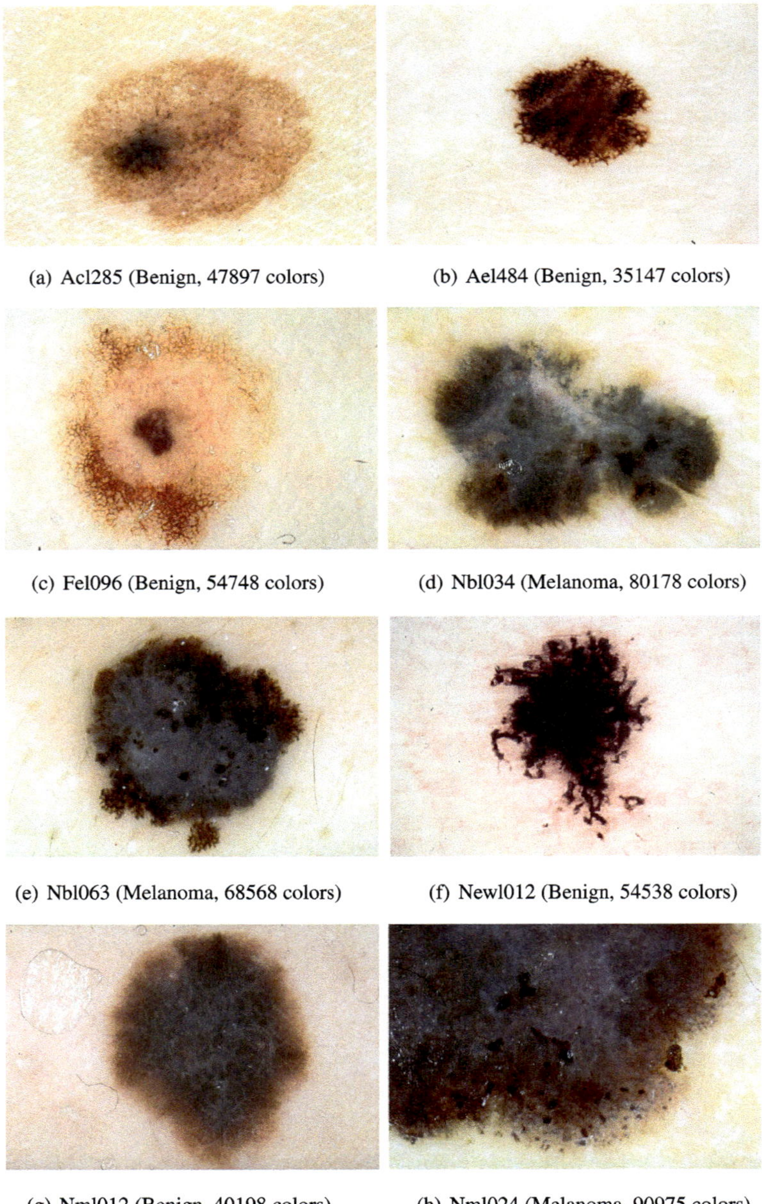

(a) Acl285 (Benign, 47897 colors)   (b) Ael484 (Benign, 35147 colors)

(c) Fel096 (Benign, 54748 colors)   (d) Nbl034 (Melanoma, 80178 colors)

(e) Nbl063 (Melanoma, 68568 colors)   (f) Newl012 (Benign, 54538 colors)

(g) Nml012 (Benign, 40198 colors)   (h) Nml024 (Melanoma, 90975 colors)

Fig. 1 Test images

3.2 Comparison of WSM Against Other Quantization Methods

The WSM method was compared to 11 well-known CQ methods:

- **Median-cut (MC)** [30]: This method starts by building a $32 \times 32 \times 32$ color histogram using 5 bits/channel uniform quantization. This histogram volume is then recursively split into smaller boxes until K boxes are obtained. At each step, the box that contains the greatest number of colors is split along the longest axis at the median point, so that the resulting subboxes each contain approximately the same number of colors. The centroids of the final K boxes are taken as the color palette.

- **Octree (OCT)** [27]: This two-phase method first builds an octree (a tree data structure in which each internal node has up to eight children) that represents the color distribution of the input image and then, starting from the bottom of the tree, prunes the tree by merging its nodes until K colors are obtained. In the experiments, the tree depth was limited to 6.

- **Variance-based method (WAN)** [65]: This method is similar to MC with the exception that at each step the box with the greatest SSE is split along the axis with the least weighted sum of projected variances at the point that minimizes the marginal squared error.

- **Greedy orthogonal bipartitioning (WU)** [68]: This method is similar to WAN with the exception that at each step the box is split along the axis that minimizes the sum of variances on both sides.

- **Center-cut (CC)** [37]: This method is similar to MC with the exception that at each step the box with the greatest range on any coordinate axis is split along its longest axis at the mean point.

- **Self-organizing map (SOM)** [17]: This method utilizes a one-dimensional self-organizing map with K neurons. A random subset of N/f pixels is used in the training phase and the final weights of the neurons are taken as the color palette. In the experiments, the highest quality configuration, i.e., $f = 1$, was used.

- **Radius-weighted mean-cut (RWM)** [75]: This method is similar to WAN with the exception that the box is split along the vector from the origin to the radius-weighted mean (rwm) at the rwm point.

- **Modified maxmin (MMM)** [70]: This method chooses the first palette color c_1 arbitrarily from the input image colors and the i-th color c_i ($i = 2, 3, \ldots, K$) is chosen to be the color that has the greatest minimum weighted $\mathcal{L}_2^2$ distance (the weights for the red, green, and blue channels are taken as 0.5, 1.0, and 0.25, respectively) to the previously selected colors, i.e., $c_1, c_2, \ldots, c_{i-1}$. Each of these initial palette colors is then recalculated as the mean of the colors assigned to it. In the experiments, the first color was chosen as the centroid of the input image colors.

- **Split and merge (SAM)** [7]: This two-phase method first partitions the color space uniformly into B partitions. This initial set of B clusters is represented as an adjacency graph. In the second phase, $(B - K)$ merge operations are performed to obtain the final K clusters. At each step of the second phase, the pair of clusters with the minimum joint quantization error are merged. In the experiments, the initial number of clusters was set to $B = 20K$.

- **Cheng and Yang (CY)** [15]: This method is similar to WAN with the exception that at each step the box is split along a specially chosen line defined by the mean color and the color that is farthest away from it at the mean point.
- **Adaptive distributing units (ADU)** [10]: This method is an adaptation of Uchiyama and Arbib's clustering algorithm [62] to CQ. ADU is a competitive learning algorithm in which units compete to represent the input point presented in each iteration. The winner is then rewarded by moving it closer to the input point at a rate of γ (the learning rate). The procedure starts with a single unit whose center is given by the centroid of the input points. New units are added by splitting existing units that reach the threshold number of wins θ until the number of units reaches K. Following [10], the algorithm parameters were set to $\theta = 400\sqrt{K}$, $t_{max} = (2K - 3)\theta$, and $\gamma = 0.015$.

The convergence of WSM was controlled by the following commonly used criterion [44]: $(SSE_{i-1} - SSE_i)/SSE_i \leq \varepsilon$, where SSE_i denotes the SSE (1) value at the end of the i-th iteration. The convergence threshold was set to $\varepsilon = 0.001$.

Tables 1, 2 and 3 compare the CQ methods with respect to MAE, MSE, and CPU time, respectively for 4, 6, and 8 colors. For the effectiveness criteria, the best (lowest) error values are shown in **bold**. It can be seen that, in general, WSM is significantly more effective than the other methods. As expected, postclustering methods are often significantly slower than the preclustering methods. Nevertheless, each CQ method requires only a few milliseconds of CPU time. Therefore, it is generally preferable to use postclustering methods that give higher quality results.

Figures 2, 3 and 4 show sample quantization results for Ael484, Nml012, and Nml024, respectively. It can be seen that, despite the small number of quantization

Table 1 MAE comparison of the quantization methods

Method	K			K		
	4	6	8	4	6	8
	Acl285			Ael484		
MC	35.7	33.2	30.2	31.6	29.7	26.0
OCT	44.5	26.3	26.6	32.2	23.6	21.3
WAN	49.4	31.5	24.6	30.5	25.6	20.5
WU	36.2	27.3	22.0	30.3	20.5	17.9
CC	51.5	32.7	31.2	34.7	23.7	20.9
SOM	36.9	26.1	23.2	33.9	24.2	22.4
RWM	35.9	25.3	22.8	31.5	21.7	17.3
MMM	43.7	34.9	25.3	29.5	20.6	19.8
SAM	35.9	31.1	30.1	29.7	26.8	25.8
CY	37.9	26.3	22.8	34.8	27.8	19.6
ADU	33.5	24.6	21.3	30.6	24.3	16.4
WSM	**33.0**	**24.5**	**19.9**	**29.1**	**19.7**	**15.9**

Table 1 (Continued)

Method	K			K		
	4	6	8	4	6	8
	Fel096			Nbl034		
MC	41.3	38.2	37.6	47.5	41.9	37.5
OCT	42.5	35.9	31.0	53.1	41.4	37.9
WAN	48.7	38.4	29.5	56.1	43.6	33.2
WU	44.0	30.4	24.5	48.1	37.1	33.1
CC	56.7	34.3	30.7	49.8	38.6	32.5
SOM	50.8	31.9	29.0	55.8	40.0	33.3
RWM	43.1	29.4	24.7	48.1	38.4	29.7
MMM	61.5	43.5	37.5	46.8	34.3	31.9
SAM	44.4	35.9	34.2	52.4	39.7	36.7
CY	43.2	31.1	27.8	50.6	37.9	30.9
ADU	**40.1**	29.4	23.1	49.5	34.4	29.0
WSM	40.3	**27.1**	**22.5**	**46.5**	**33.6**	**28.4**
	Nbl063			Newl012		
MC	54.9	41.8	39.2	36.8	34.8	31.9
OCT	55.2	38.4	30.4	36.7	26.6	24.9
WAN	53.7	38.0	32.5	40.9	32.6	29.2
WU	44.0	36.3	28.6	37.2	28.5	24.1
CC	44.9	37.2	31.9	40.8	31.2	30.0
SOM	62.1	37.0	31.0	43.3	30.9	27.0
RWM	44.7	38.4	28.1	38.0	28.3	24.1
MMM	46.0	**33.4**	30.5	**35.4**	31.1	29.1
SAM	55.7	45.4	42.4	39.9	35.3	34.8
CY	50.3	36.5	29.7	39.9	31.0	26.4
ADU	44.9	34.7	27.3	35.8	**26.3**	**22.2**
WSM	**43.7**	35.8	**26.8**	35.6	26.4	22.4
	Nml012			Nml024		
MC	46.3	31.2	27.8	56.2	43.0	41.6
OCT	45.1	39.6	29.9	52.5	43.8	39.8
WAN	51.6	35.5	25.6	56.8	45.8	36.3
WU	38.1	27.4	22.7	52.6	38.8	32.4
CC	42.3	34.0	27.0	52.0	45.8	37.6
SOM	56.5	35.7	23.9	52.4	47.7	34.9
RWM	38.9	28.5	24.1	50.9	39.2	33.8
MMM	39.4	32.9	27.0	54.3	40.7	35.0
SAM	38.3	32.4	30.9	52.8	38.8	34.1
CY	46.6	29.6	25.5	56.3	42.2	32.8
ADU	45.6	28.2	22.0	53.0	38.5	32.9
WSM	**37.1**	**26.3**	**21.5**	**50.5**	**37.2**	**31.6**

Table 2 MSE comparison of the quantization methods

Method	K			K		
	4	6	8	4	6	8
	Ac1285			Ae1484		
MC	759.1	639.1	526.1	625.9	524.6	379.5
OCT	1750.7	438.0	435.6	685.0	521.8	424.1
WAN	1652.2	647.0	416.1	751.9	497.9	335.2
WU	786.7	477.6	283.7	598.6	295.3	228.6
CC	1496.3	605.2	560.3	693.6	382.9	300.3
SOM	895.8	467.0	415.7	1325.4	594.0	552.0
RWM	774.4	421.1	298.3	639.3	375.3	190.8
MMM	1077.7	668.3	372.5	586.2	267.7	246.7
SAM	869.0	578.0	548.2	589.1	423.0	391.7
CY	823.9	433.6	329.5	684.2	410.9	234.9
ADU	718.8	406.7	297.1	1070.9	685.3	240.4
WSM	**714.6**	**359.8**	**234.5**	**522.8**	**256.5**	**173.5**
	Fe1096			Nb1034		
MC	945.4	787.5	762.8	1177.3	939.8	761.7
OCT	1351.6	678.6	546.3	1829.2	970.2	844.0
WAN	1884.7	909.5	559.6	1771.9	1093.7	658.2
WU	1182.1	540.4	380.1	1249.0	779.9	628.2
CC	1654.5	637.3	503.4	1313.0	833.3	568.8
SOM	2151.3	1039.4	853.9	1850.3	1004.0	696.9
RWM	1039.1	522.2	341.3	1196.1	805.3	514.0
MMM	2018.6	946.7	716.3	1211.9	674.1	594.9
SAM	1249.6	712.2	659.9	1561.4	890.2	768.9
CY	1027.1	572.3	424.5	1325.0	777.6	533.1
ADU	1329.8	491.9	334.2	1242.5	648.3	476.3
WSM	**884.4**	**436.8**	**313.1**	**1147.0**	**637.0**	**458.9**
	Nb1063			New1012		
MC	1610.4	892.2	791.0	770.5	655.8	528.9
OCT	1806.2	881.3	504.5	766.0	400.3	354.4
WAN	1585.2	880.8	602.9	1112.6	684.1	534.9
WU	1086.0	751.0	509.9	776.1	477.7	354.0
CC	1138.7	784.5	556.5	910.2	522.8	478.2
SOM	2268.2	787.8	608.4	1883.6	769.0	649.4
RWM	1098.2	794.7	459.0	781.9	464.3	313.1
MMM	1156.0	**635.6**	521.0	754.1	522.2	436.6
SAM	1611.6	1084.0	972.0	1012.0	732.3	709.5
CY	1283.6	708.1	486.5	852.7	567.5	381.0

Table 2 (Continued)

Method	K			K		
	4	6	8	4	6	8
ADU	1085.8	674.9	457.3	1000.4	409.2	310.2
WSM	**1062.2**	726.2	**405.4**	**726.6**	**393.8**	**281.8**
	Nml012			Nml024		
MC	1400.2	520.0	418.4	1761.6	1016.2	960.7
OCT	1431.2	1268.0	582.2	1515.5	1018.0	844.4
WAN	1552.9	736.2	410.6	1821.5	1170.0	774.8
WU	922.6	458.0	306.8	1444.3	825.2	592.9
CC	1055.3	729.9	433.9	1454.8	1153.5	852.3
SOM	1924.2	1029.5	376.5	1448.9	1311.9	772.8
RWM	880.3	447.1	330.5	1354.7	841.9	630.7
MMM	971.8	640.7	395.8	1524.9	907.7	673.1
SAM	849.7	606.7	561.9	1572.7	839.4	646.3
CY	1331.8	479.9	371.0	1735.5	956.7	561.0
ADU	1133.4	466.7	292.1	1443.2	789.0	587.5
WSM	**789.1**	**412.8**	**274.3**	**1316.6**	**763.7**	**550.7**

Table 3 CPU time comparison of the quantization methods

Method	K			K		
	4	6	8	4	6	8
	Acl285			Ael484		
MC	0.1	0.0	0.0	0.0	0.0	0.0
OCT	40.8	40.7	41.1	31.3	40.5	40.8
WAN	0.2	0.2	0.2	0.0	0.2	0.4
WU	0.1	0.8	1.6	0.1	1.1	0.6
CC	5.6	6.6	7.7	5.6	7.1	6.8
SOM	21.5	30.9	40.1	20.7	34.6	41.6
RWM	4.8	5.7	5.7	4.2	6.1	6.2
MMM	20.7	22.5	24.6	17.2	19.5	19.7
SAM	0.7	0.8	0.8	0.1	0.1	0.3
CY	4.0	6.2	6.5	4.3	5.5	5.8
ADU	0.3	0.6	0.8	0.3	0.1	0.9
WSM	19.9	25.4	19.0	11.3	15.0	18.2
	Fel096			Nbl034		
MC	0.1	0.0	0.0	0.0	0.0	0.0
OCT	40.8	43.4	42.4	43.9	50.1	50.7

M.E. Celebi et al.

Table 3 (Continued)

Method	K			K		
	4	6	8	4	6	8
WAN	0.0	0.3	0.6	0.0	0.0	0.1
WU	0.3	0.9	0.6	0.2	0.4	1.0
CC	4.8	6.4	8.3	5.4	8.4	8.6
SOM	21.7	32.4	40.2	20.1	30.7	40.2
RWM	4.2	5.2	6.3	4.4	7.5	7.2
MMM	20.3	22.9	25.2	29.7	39.7	40.8
SAM	0.8	0.7	0.5	0.6	0.8	0.7
CY	4.4	7.4	7.1	5.2	5.2	7.5
ADU	0.3	0.1	0.7	0.0	0.6	0.7
WSM	20.5	20.1	18.0	20.6	29.8	27.4
	Nbl063			Newl012		
MC	0.0	0.0	0.0	0.0	0.0	0.0
OCT	41.2	48.2	46.7	37.8	42.2	43.8
WAN	0.0	0.2	0.2	0.2	0.1	0.3
WU	0.3	0.5	0.7	0.6	0.7	1.5
CC	6.0	7.6	8.6	5.5	7.4	7.2
SOM	20.3	31.8	39.7	25.2	36.6	41.0
RWM	4.7	5.8	6.4	4.3	6.4	7.9
MMM	24.8	31.0	32.9	23.7	27.1	28.3
SAM	0.2	0.5	0.9	0.4	0.6	0.4
CY	4.8	6.4	7.3	5.0	5.4	8.7
ADU	0.1	0.7	0.7	0.2	0.7	1.0
WSM	15.1	18.8	24.3	20.1	20.0	21.1
	Nml012			Nml024		
MC	0.0	0.0	0.0	0.0	0.0	0.0
OCT	40.4	41.3	47.2	47.0	52.1	54.8
WAN	0.1	0.2	0.4	0.2	0.2	0.5
WU	0.7	1.2	1.3	0.9	1.2	0.8
CC	4.8	7.8	8.4	7.5	9.8	11.3
SOM	21.8	33.1	40.1	22.0	35.2	40.2
RWM	4.8	5.6	6.0	5.9	8.8	11.6
MMM	19.7	20.8	21.0	41.5	44.0	46.3
SAM	0.3	0.8	0.5	0.5	0.5	0.6
CY	5.1	5.9	6.2	6.3	9.5	9.4
ADU	0.3	0.5	1.0	0.3	0.6	0.9
WSM	20.0	16.5	20.3	21.0	24.5	24.5

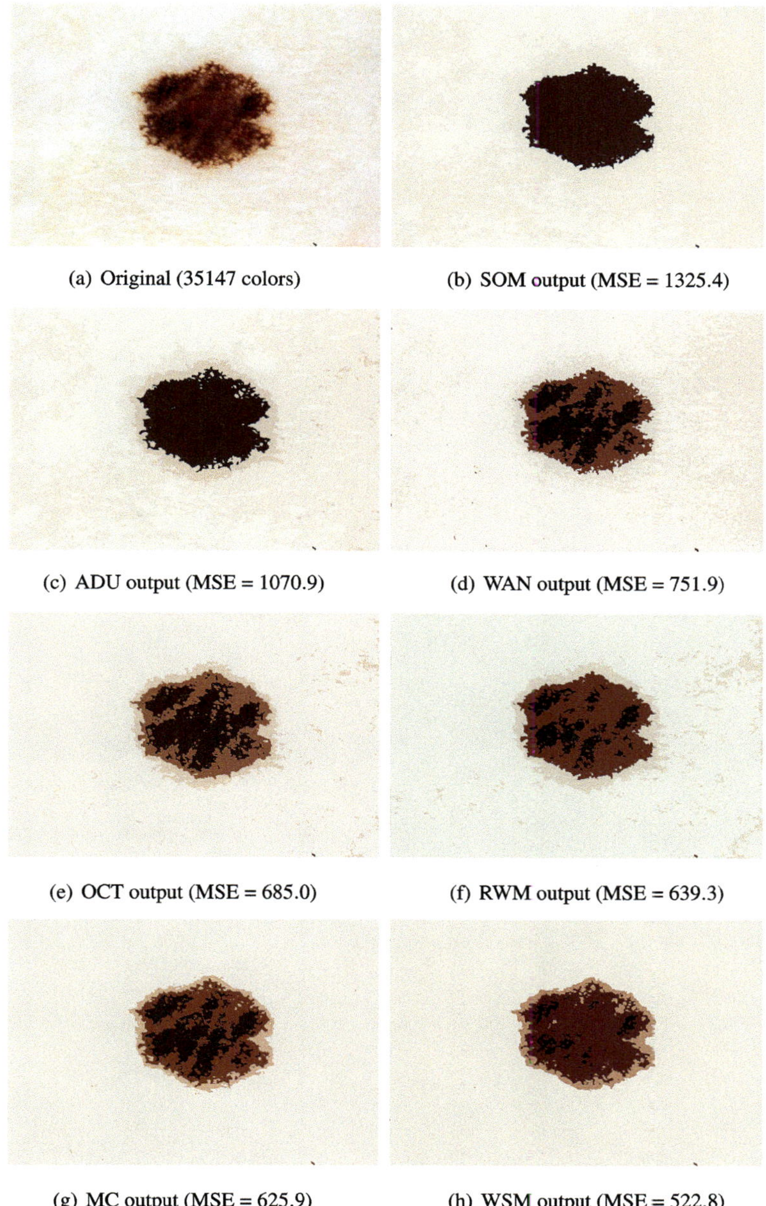

(a) Original (35147 colors)

(b) SOM output (MSE = 1325.4)

(c) ADU output (MSE = 1070.9)

(d) WAN output (MSE = 751.9)

(e) OCT output (MSE = 685.0)

(f) RWM output (MSE = 639.3)

(g) MC output (MSE = 625.9)

(h) WSM output (MSE = 522.8)

Fig. 2 Ael484 quantized to $K = 4$ colors

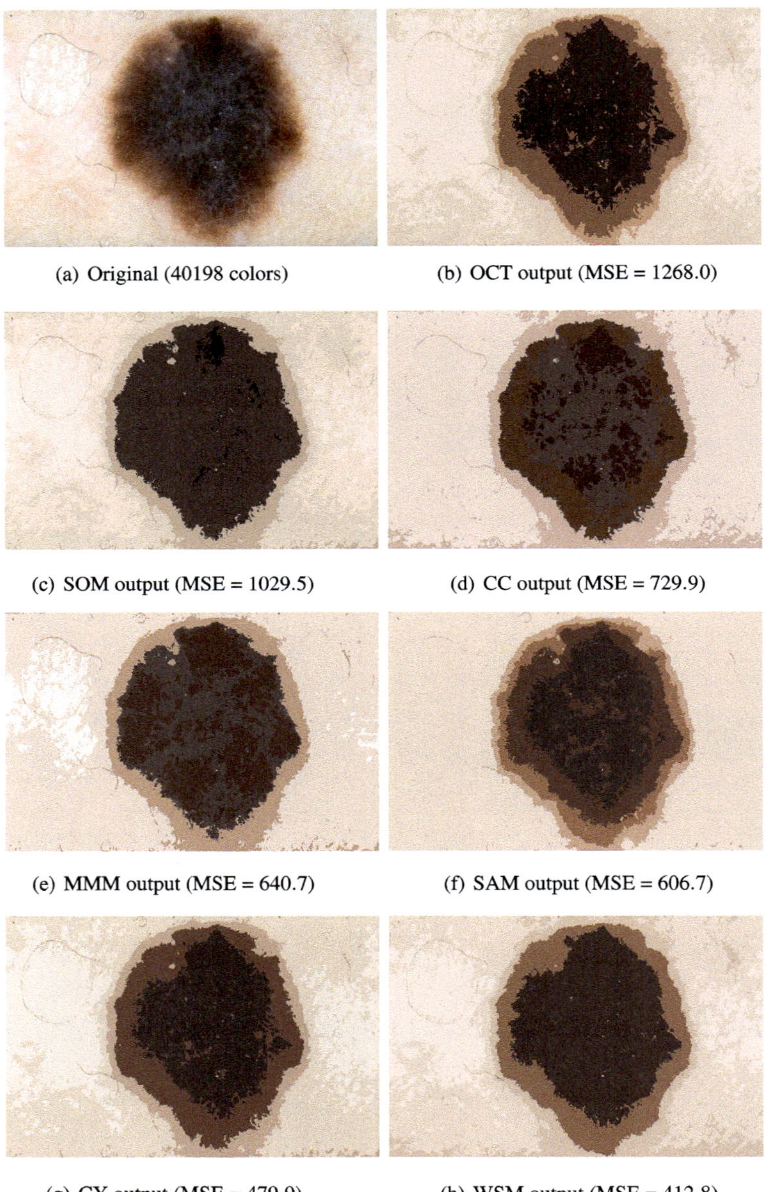

(a) Original (40198 colors)

(b) OCT output (MSE = 1268.0)

(c) SOM output (MSE = 1029.5)

(d) CC output (MSE = 729.9)

(e) MMM output (MSE = 640.7)

(f) SAM output (MSE = 606.7)

(g) CY output (MSE = 479.9)

(h) WSM output (MSE = 412.8)

Fig. 3 Nml012 quantized to $K = 6$ colors

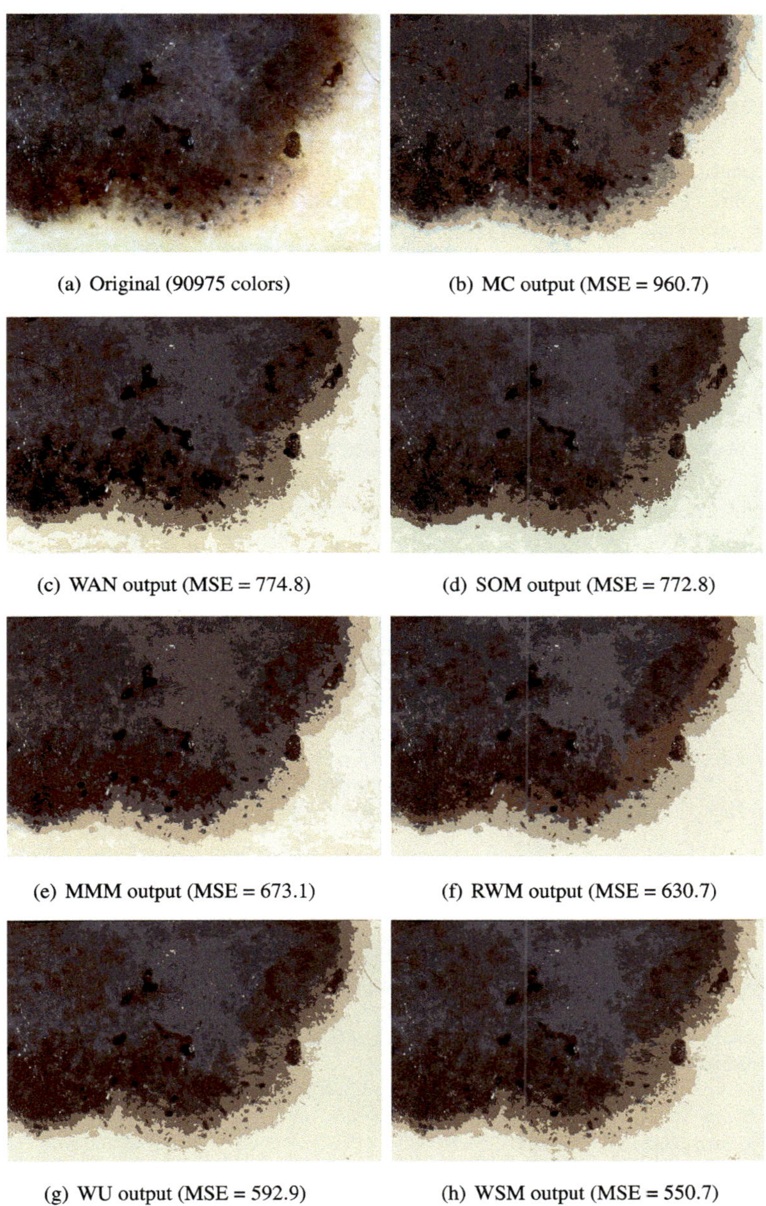

(a) Original (90975 colors)   (b) MC output (MSE = 960.7)

(c) WAN output (MSE = 774.8)   (d) SOM output (MSE = 772.8)

(e) MMM output (MSE = 673.1)   (f) RWM output (MSE = 630.7)

(g) WU output (MSE = 592.9)   (h) WSM output (MSE = 550.7)

Fig. 4 Nml024 quantized to $K = 8$ colors

levels used, WSM performs exceptionally well in allocating representative colors to various regions of the images.

4 Conclusions and Future Work

In this paper, we investigated the applicability of a recently proposed k-means based CQ method to dermoscopy image quantization. This method improves upon the conventional k-means based CQ method by using data reduction, sample weighting, accelerated nearest neighbor search, and deterministic cluster center initialization. Extensive experiments on a diverse set of dermoscopy images demonstrated that the proposed method outperforms state-of-the-art quantization methods with respect to distortion minimization. Other advantages of the presented method include ease of implementation, very high computational speed, and the possibility of incorporating spatial information into the quantization procedure.

The proposed method can be readily utilized to improve color based similarity retrieval of dermoscopy images. It can also be used to facilitate the detection of skin lesion borders by simplifying the images prior to segmentation. The presence of multiple colors (white, red, light brown, dark brown, blue-gray, and black) in a skin lesion is a highly significant feature of invasive melanoma. Melanomas are usually characterized by three or more colors, and in about 40% of them even five or six colors are present [2]. Our method can be combined with a suitable cluster validity measure to determine the number of dominant colors in a skin lesion, which is potentially useful for diagnostic purposes.

Acknowledgements   This publication was made possible by grants from the Louisiana Board of Regents (LEQSF2008-11-RD-A-12), US National Science Foundation (0959583, 1117457), and National Natural Science Foundation of China (61050110449, 61073120).

References

1. Aloise D, Deshpande A, Hansen P, Popat P (2009) NP-hardness of Euclidean sum-of-squares clustering. Mach Learn 75(2):245–248
2. Argenziano G, Soyer H, De Giorgi V et al (2002) Dermoscopy: a tutorial. EDRA Medical Publishing & New Media, Milan
3. Balasubramanian R, Allebach J (1991) A new approach to palette selection for color images. J Imaging Technol 17(6):284–290
4. Balasubramanian R, Bouman C, Allebach J (1994) Sequential scalar quantization of color images. J Electron Imaging 3(1):45–59
5. Bing Z, Junyi S, Qinke P (2004) An adjustable algorithm for color quantization. Pattern Recognit Lett 25(16):1787–1797
6. Bottou L, Bengio Y (1995) Convergence properties of the K-means algorithms. In: Advances in neural information processing systems, vol 7. MIT Press, Cambridge, pp 585–592
7. Brun L, Mokhtari M (2000) Two high speed color quantization algorithms. In: Proceedings of the 1st international conference on color in graphics and image processing, pp 116–121

8. Brun L, Trémeau A (2002) Color quantization. In: Digital color imaging handbook. CRC Press, Boca Raton, pp 589–638

9. Cak S, Dizdar EN, Ersak A (1998) A fuzzy colour quantizer for renderers. Displays 19(2):61–65

10. Celebi ME (2009) An effective color quantization method based on the competitive learning paradigm. In: Proceedings of the international conference on image processing, computer vision, and pattern recognition, vol 2, pp 876–880

11. Celebi ME (2011) Improving the performance of K-means for color quantization. Image Vis Comput 29(4):260–271

12. Celebi ME, Kingravi H, Celiker F (2010) Fast color space transformations using minimax approximations. IET Image Process 4(2):70–80

13. Celebi ME, Schaefer G (2010) Neural gas clustering for color reduction. In: Proceedings of the international conference on image processing, computer vision, and pattern recognition, pp 429–432

14. Chang CH, Xu P, Xiao R, Srikanthan T (2005) New adaptive color quantization method based on self-organizing maps. IEEE Trans Neural Netw 16(1):237–249

15. Cheng S, Yang C (2001) Fast and novel technique for color quantization using reduction of color space dimensionality. Pattern Recognit Lett 22(8):845–856

16. Chung KL, Huang YH, Wang JP, Cheng MS (2012) Speedup of color palette indexing in self-organization of Kohonen feature map. Expert Syst Appl 39(3):2427–2432

17. Dekker A (1994) Kohonen neural networks for optimal colour quantization. Netw: Comput Neural Syst 5(3):351–367

18. Deng Y, Manjunath B (2001) Unsupervised segmentation of color-texture regions in images and video. IEEE Trans Pattern Anal Mach Intell 23(8):800–810

19. Deng Y, Manjunath B, Kenney C, Moore M, Shin H (2001) An efficient color representation for image retrieval. IEEE Trans Image Process 10(1):140–147

20. Elkan C (2003) Using the triangle inequality to accelerate K-means. In: Proceedings of the 20th international conference on machine learning, pp 147–153

21. Equitz WH (1989) A new vector quantization clustering algorithm. IEEE Trans Acoust Speech Signal Process 37(10):1568–1575

22. Fletcher P (1991) A SIMD parallel colour quantization algorithm. Comput Graph 15(3):365–373

23. Frackiewicz M, Palus H (2011) KM and KHM clustering techniques for colour image quantisation. In: Computational vision and medical image processing: recent trends. Springer, Berlin, pp 161–174

24. Fränti P, Virmajoki O, Hautamäki V (2006) Fast agglomerative clustering using a k-nearest neighbor graph. IEEE Trans Pattern Anal Mach Intell 28(11):1875–1881

25. Gan G, Ma C, Wu J (2007) Data clustering: theory, algorithms, and applications. SIAM, Philadelphia

26. Gentile RS, Allebach JP, Walowit E (1990) Quantization of color images based on uniform color spaces. J Imaging Technol 16(1):11–21

27. Gervautz M, Purgathofer W (1988) A simple method for color quantization: octree quantization. In: New trends in computer graphics. Springer, Berlin, pp 219–231

28. Goldberg N (1991) Colour image quantization for high resolution graphics display. Image Vis Comput 9(5):303–312

29. Hamerly G (2010) Making k-means even faster. In: Proceedings of the 2010 SIAM international conference on data mining, pp 130–140

30. Heckbert P (1982) Color image quantization for frame buffer display. ACM SIGGRAPH Comput Graph 16(3):297–307

31. Hsieh IS, Fan KC (2000) An adaptive clustering algorithm for color quantization. Pattern Recognit Lett 21(4):337–346

32. Hu YC, Lee MG (2007) K-means based color palette design scheme with the use of stable flags. J Electron Imaging 16(3):033,003

33. Hu YC, Su BH (2008) Accelerated K-means clustering algorithm for colour image quantization. Imaging Sci J 56(1):29–40
34. Hu YC, Su BH (2008) Accelerated pixel mapping scheme for colour image quantisation. Imaging Sci J 56(2):68–78
35. Huang YL, Chang RF (2004) A fast finite-state algorithm for generating RGB palettes of color quantized images. J Inf Sci Eng 20(4):771–782
36. Jin X, Kim S, Han J, Cao L, Yin Z (2009) GAD: general activity detection for fast clustering on large data. In: Proceedings of the 2009 SIAM international conference on data mining, pp 2–13
37. Joy G, Xiang Z (1993) Center-cut for color image quantization. Vis Comput 10(1):62–66
38. Kanjanawanishkul K, Uyyanonvara B (2005) Novel fast color reduction algorithm for time-constrained applications. J Vis Commun Image Represent 16(3):311–332
39. Kanungo T, Mount D, Netanyahu N, Piatko C, Silverman R, Wu A (2002) An efficient K-means clustering algorithm: analysis and implementation. IEEE Trans Pattern Anal Mach Intell 24(7):881–892
40. Kasuga H, Yamamoto H, Okamoto M (2000) Color quantization using the fast K-means algorithm. Syst Comput Jpn 31(8):33–40
41. Kim DW, Lee K, Lee D (2004) A novel initialization scheme for the fuzzy c-means algorithm for color clustering. Pattern Recognit Lett 25(2):227–237
42. Kuo CT, Cheng SC (2007) Fusion of color edge detection and color quantization for color image watermarking using principal axes analysis. Pattern Recognit 40(12):3691–3704
43. Lai J, Liaw YC (2008) Improvement of the K-means clustering filtering algorithm. Pattern Recognit 41(12):3677–3681
44. Linde Y, Buzo A, Gray R (1980) An algorithm for vector quantizer design. IEEE Trans Commun 28(1):84–95
45. Lloyd S (1982) Least squares quantization in PCM. IEEE Trans Inf Theory 28(2):129–136
46. Lo K, Chan Y, Yu M (2003) Colour quantization by three-dimensional frequency diffusion. Pattern Recognit Lett 24(14):2325–2334
47. Mahajan M, Nimbhorkar P, Varadarajan K (2012) The planar k-means problem is NP-hard. Theor Comput Sci 442:13–21
48. Mojsilovic A, Soljanin E (2001) Color quantization and processing by Fibonacci lattices. IEEE Trans Image Process 10(11):1712–1725
49. Orchard M, Bouman C (1991) Color quantization of images. IEEE Trans Signal Process 39(12):2677–2690
50. Ozdemir D, Akarun L (2002) Fuzzy algorithm for color quantization of images. Pattern Recognit 35(8):1785–1791
51. Papamarkos N, Atsalakis A, Strouthopoulos C (2002) Adaptive color reduction. IEEE Trans Syst, Man, Cybern Part B 32(1):44–56
52. Phillips S (2002) Acceleration of K-means and related clustering algorithms. In: Proceedings of the 4th international workshop on algorithm engineering and experiments, pp 166–177
53. Rasti J, Monadjemi A, Vafaei A (2011) Color reduction using a multi-stage Kohonen self-organizing map with redundant features. Expert Syst Appl 38(10):13,188–13,197
54. Schaefer G (2011) Intelligent approaches to colour palette design. In: Innovations in intelligent image analysis. Springer, Berlin, pp 275–289
55. Schaefer G, Zhou H (2009) Fuzzy clustering for colour reduction in images. Telecommun Syst 40(1–2):17–25
56. Schaefer G, Zhou H, Celebi ME, Hassanien AE (2011) Rough colour quantisation. Int J Hybrid Intell Syst 8(1):25–30
57. Scheunders P (1997) Comparison of clustering algorithms applied to color image quantization. Pattern Recognit Lett 18(11–13):1379–1384
58. Selim SZ, Ismail MA (1984) K-means-type algorithms: a generalized convergence theorem and characterization of local optimality. IEEE Trans Pattern Anal Mach Intell 6(1):81–87

59. Sertel O, Kong J, Catalyurek UV, Lozanski G, Saltz JH, Gurcan MN (2009) Histopathological image analysis using model-based intermediate representations and color texture: follicular lymphoma grading. J Signal Process Syst 55(1–3):169–183
60. Sherkat N, Allen T, Wong S (2005) Use of colour for hand-filled form analysis and recognition. Pattern Anal Appl 8(1):163–180
61. Sirisathitkul Y, Auwatanamongkol S, Uyyanonvara B (2004) Color image quantization using distances between adjacent colors along the color axis with highest color variance. Pattern Recognit Lett 25(9):1025–1043
62. Uchiyama T, Arbib M (1994) An algorithm for competitive learning in clustering problems. Pattern Recognit 27(10):1415–1421
63. Velho L, Gomez J, Sobreiro MVR (1997) Color image quantization by pairwise clustering. In: Proceedings of the 10th Brazilian symposium on computer graphics and image processing, pp 203–210
64. Verevka O, Buchanan J (1995) Local K-means algorithm for colour image quantization. In: Proceedings of the graphics/vision interface conference, pp 128–135
65. Wan SJ, Wong SKM, Prusinkiewicz P (1990) Variance-based color image quantization for frame buffer display. Color Res Appl 15:52–58
66. Wang S, Cai K, Lu J, Liu X, Wu E (2010) Real-time coherent stylization for augmented reality. Vis Comput 26(6–8):445–455
67. Wen Q, Celebi ME (2011) Hard vs. fuzzy C-means clustering for color quantization. EURASIP J Adv Signal Process 2011(1):118–129
68. Wu X (1991) Efficient statistical computations for optimal color quantization. In: Graphics gems, vol II. Academic Press, New York, pp 126–133
69. Wu X (1992) Color quantization by dynamic programming and principal analysis. ACM Trans Graph 11(4):348–372
70. Xiang Z (1997) Color image quantization by minimizing the maximum intercluster distance. ACM Trans Graph 16(3):260–276
71. Xiang Z (2007) Color quantization. In: Handbook of approximation algorithms and meta-heuristics. Chapman & Hall/CRC, London, pp 86-1–86-17
72. Xiang Z, Joy G (1994) Color image quantization by agglomerative clustering. IEEE Comput Graph Appl 14(3):44–48
73. Xiao Y, Leung CS, Lam PM, Ho TY (2012) Self-organizing map-based color palette for high-dynamic range texture compression. Neural Comput Appl 21(4):639–647
74. Yang CK, Tsai WH (1998) Color image compression using quantization, thresholding, and edge detection techniques all based on the moment-preserving principle. Pattern Recognit Lett 19(2):205–215
75. Yang CY, Lin JC (1996) RWM-cut for color image quantization. Comput Graph 20(4):577–588

Grading the Severity of Diabetic Macular Edema Cases Based on Color Eye Fundus Images

Daniel Welfer, Jacob Scharcanski, Pablo Gautério Cavalcanti,
Diane Ruschel Marinho, Laura W.B. Ludwig, Cleyson M. Kitamura,
and Melissa M. Dal Pizzol

Abstract Current computer-aided diagnosis (CAD) systems tend to neglect the detection and grading of Diabetic Macular Edema (DME) signs. This chapter introduces a new computer based scheme for detecting and grading DME signs using color eye fundus images. The grading scheme integrates methods for: (a) detecting retinal structures (e.g. optic disk and fovea); (b) detecting lesions in the retina (e.g. exudates); (c) analyzing the spatial distribution of DME signs in the retina; and (d) grading the severity of a DME case as *absent*, *mild*, *moderate* or *severe*. In a preliminary experimental evaluation of our DME grading scheme using publicly avail-

D. Welfer (✉)
UNIPAMPA, Federal University of Pampa, Av. Tiarajú 810, CEP. 97546-550, Alegrete, RS, Brasil
e-mail: danielwelfer@unipampa.edu.br

J. Scharcanski · P.G. Cavalcanti
Institute of Informatics, Federal University of Rio Grande do Sul. Av. Bento Gonçalves 9500,
CEP. 91509-900, Porto Alegre, RS, Brasil

J. Scharcanski
e-mail: jacobs@inf.ufrgs.br

P.G. Cavalcanti
e-mail: pgcavalcanti@inf.ufrgs.br

D.R. Marinho
Faculty of Medicine, Federal University of Rio Grande do Sul, Rua Ramiro Barcelos, 2400, CEP.
90035-003, Porto Alegre, RS, Brasil
e-mail: diane@portoweb.com.br

L.W.B. Ludwig · C.M. Kitamura · M.M. Dal Pizzol
Hospital de Clinicas de Porto Alegre, Rua Ramiro Barcelos, 2350, CEP. 90035-903, Porto Alegre,
RS, Brasil

L.W.B. Ludwig
e-mail: laludwig@hotmail.com

C.M. Kitamura
e-mail: cmk_@hotmail.com

M.M. Dal Pizzol
e-mail: melissa.olhos@via-rs.net

M.E. Celebi, G. Schaefer (eds.), *Color Medical Image Analysis*,
Lecture Notes in Computational Vision and Biomechanics 6,
DOI 10.1007/978-94-007-5389-1_6, © Springer Science+Business Media Dordrecht 2013

able eye fundus images (i.e., DIARETDB1 image database), an accuracy of 94.29 % was obtained with respect to the mode of the evaluations of the same DME cases by four experts. This is encouraging, since a similar DME grading performance is achieved by a DME expert. In order to calculate the clinicians grading performance, we assumed the mode of all experts DME gradings as the reference evaluation for each case. Thus, if an expert assigned each DME case to the class identified as the mode of the experts severity gradings, that expert achieved an accuracy of 100 %.

1 Introduction

DME has three severity levels [2, 22], namely: (1) DME mild; (2) DME moderate; (3) DME severe. Mild DME is usually characterized by retinal thickening or hard exudates occurring far from the macula center. Moderate DME is characterized by the occurrence of retinal thickening or by hard exudates in the neighborhood of the macula center. Finally, severe DME presents retinal thickening or hard exudates near the macula center. Exudates are aggregates of leaked fatty material, formed by the precipitation of blood products (e.g. lipids and protein) in the retina, choroid or optic disk, and often appear as bright yellow lesions in eye fundus images. The detection of hard exudates provides insufficient information to grade the Diabetic Macular Edema (DME), since the spatial distribution of the exudates with respect to the macula center is very important. The macula center is very important in terms of visual acuity because it is densely populated by cones, the color receptors of the visual system. For instance, exudates covering a larger area, but far from the macula center can be the less harmful to the patient visual acuity than exudates covering a smaller area near the macula center [10]. The further away from the macular region, less severe is the Diabetic Macular Edema.

In most eye fundus images, the macula appears as the darker image region, and its central portion is called the fovea. Physically, the fovea is a circle with of approximately 0.25 mm of diameter [17], and its center is located on the temporal side of the optic nerve, at a number of optic disk diameters from the optic disk center [10] (e.g. 2 disk diameters). The temporal side is the side opposite to the optic disk (e.g. if the optic disk is in the left side, the temporal side is in the right side). Thus, optic disk parameters (like its diameter) are important for detecting other retinal structures, such as the fovea. Moreover, the detecting the optic disk helps to avoid the detection of exudate false positives (i.e. since the optic disk may be bright yellow and can be confused with exudates). Figure 1 illustrates a typical fundus image, and some important retinal features, like the fovea, the blood vessels arcade, the optic disk and exudate lesions. Therefore, grading the Diabetic Macular Edema in color eye fundus images can be done efficiently if the optic disk and the fovea are located first, and then the spatial distribution of the exudates is evaluated around the fovea center (see Fig. 1).

In this chapter, we present a computer-aided scheme for grading the Diabetic Macular Edema. As proposed by Lalonde et al. [15], our scheme has two main steps,

Fig. 1 Main features and exudate lesions on a typical truecolor red-green-blue (RGB) fundus image

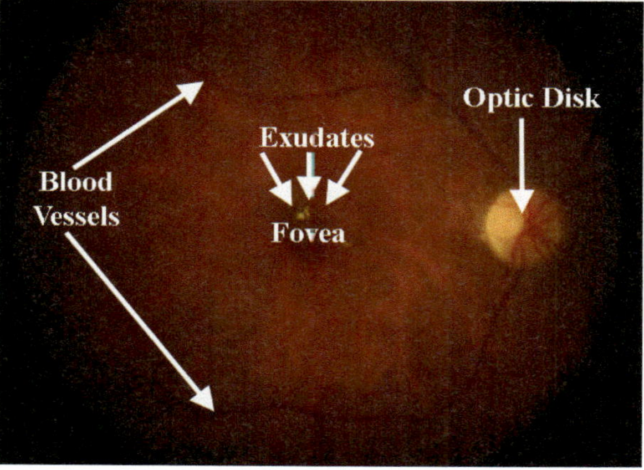

namely: (1) detection of retina structures and lesion signs; and (2) evaluation of lesions signs. These steps are detailed in the next sections. This work is organized as follows. Recent advances in computer-aided diagnosis (CAD) and related systems are discussed in Sect. 2. Section 3 describes the data used to evaluate the components of our grading scheme, and details our DME grading scheme in Sect. 3.1. Experimental results are presented and discussed in Sect. 4, and our conclusions and ideas for future work are presented in Sect. 5.

2 Related Work

Hayashi et al. [6] presented a CAD system to detect vessel tree abnormalities on eye fundus images, without focusing on DME issues. Goh et al. [5] proposed a diabetic retinal image screening system for classifying retinas as normal/abnormal. Their system detects the optic disk, exudates and retina vessels, but it can not detect the fovea or grade DME cases. Lalonde et al. [9], proposed a system for automatically detecting retinal lesions (e.g. microaneurysms and exudates) and other anatomical structures (e.g. optic disk and macula). Their system can register fundus images, but it was not designed to account for the spatial distribution of exudates near the fovea center, consequently it is not able to grade DME. Simandjuntak et al. [15] designed a CAD system for detecting structures like the optic disk, macula, blood vessels and microaneurysms. Their ultimate goal is to detect diabetic retinopathies in their early stages based only on the detected microaneurysms. However, they are not concerned with DME, since the detection of exudate lesions and their distribution around the fovea center are not computed. Yen et al. [23] proposed to grade diabetic retinopathies on fundus images using a hybrid intelligent system to detect the signs of non proliferative diabetic retinopathies (NPDR). Nevertheless, their method can not evaluate DME and its evolution.

Li et al. [10] proposed methods for the automatic detection of features in retinal images. First, they detect the optic disk using principal components analysis (PCA),

Table 1 Some major features of the proposed method and of other CAD schemes available in the literature

Methods	Provides the detection of anatomical structures in the retina	Provides the detection of lesions signs in the retina	Provides an analysis of the lesion distribution	Able to grade DME cases
Hayashi et al. [6]	Yes	No	No	No
Goh et al. [5]	Yes	Yes	No	No
Lalonde et al. [9]	Yes	Yes	No	No
Simandjuntak et al. [15]	Yes	Yes	No	No
Yen et al. [23]	Yes	Yes	No	No
Li et al. [10]	Yes	Yes	Yes	No
Walter et al. [18]	Yes	Yes	No	No
Sopharak et al. [16]	Yes	Yes	No	No
Our proposed method	Yes	Yes	Yes	Yes

and then they define the fovea region as a circle located a number of optic disk diameters away from the optic disk center, in the temporal side of the optic disk. Although they presented an analysis of the spatial distribution of exudates around the fovea center, they did not show an extensive evaluation of their method, neither how to use it for grading DME.

CAD system based on mathematical morphology also have been proposed for different applications. Walter et al. [18] proposed a method based on a sliding window to detect exudates. First, a morphological closing operator is used to remove the retinal vessels, and then a sliding window returns the local gray level variability in the vicinity of each pixel, which is used to detect exudate candidates. Afterwards, morphological reconstruction is used to detect the exudate lesions more accurately. All exudates in the optic disk region are eliminated to reduce false positives, since both, the exudates and the optic disk, can have similar brightness and shape. However, Walter et al. method do not consider the spatial distribution of exudates around the macula center, consequently DME grading is not performed. Also, Sopharak et al. [16] proposed a method similar to the approach of Walter et al. [18]. First, they segment and exclude the optic disk to avoid false positives. Afterwards, they detect exudate lesions. Their method for detecting exudates is based on morphological operations and the local variability image. Their approach also detects the macular region in order to describe the distribution of the exudates around the macula center. However, the analysis of the distribution of exudate lesions around the fovea center was not presented. Table 1 summarizes the major features of the proposed method and of other CAD systems available in the literature.

In this chapter, we present our grading scheme for detecting and grading signs of Diabetic Macular Edema (DME) in color eye fundus images. Since we did not find other approaches focused specifically on this theme, we believe that our contribution innovates in this area.

3 Materials and Methods

We used in our experiments 89 color eye fundus images of the DIARETDB1 [8]. The DIARETDB1 database is available on the WEB, and consists of a total of 89 color eye fundus images of 1500×1152 pixels at 24 bit RGB, captured using a $50°$ field-of-view digital fundus camera. In the DIARETDB1 database, there are 47 retinal images containing hard exudates, and 42 without hard exudates lesions. These images vary in quality (i.e. uneven background illumination). In some cases, images without hard exudates contain signs of another lesions such as microaneurysms and hemorrhages [8].

However, it shall be observed that two types of references were used in this work (i.e. ground truth), namely: (1) reference images for the retinal structures and lesions; and (2) references for the Diabetic Macular Edema stages. In the first case, each image was marked by four ophthalmologists. Afterwards, the mean contour (i.e. the average contour of the marked retinal structures and lesions signs) was calculated for each image of DIARETDB1, and then it was used as a ground truth image. In the second case, the Diabetic Macular Edema stage of each DIARETDB1 image was evaluated by four ophthalmologists. Afterwards, for each DIARETDB1 image, the Diabetic Macular Edema stage most frequently diagnosed by the experts was computed (i.e. the mode of the DME stage diagnoses). Next, the mode of the Diabetic Macular Edema stage evaluations for each DIARETDB1 image was used as the reference (i.e. ground truth), and the experts evaluation performances are calculated with respect to this reference.

3.1 The Computer-Aided DME Grading Scheme

The grading scheme has two steps namely: (1) Detection of retina structures and lesion signs; (2) Prescreening of lesions signs. In the following sections we describe in detail all methods comprising each step.

3.2 Detection of Retina Structures and Lesion Signs

In this section, we detail our automated methods developed for detecting: (a) optic disk (see Sect. 3.2.1); (b) fovea center (see Sect. 3.2.2); and exudate lesions (see Sect. 3.2.3).

3.2.1 Detecting the Optic Disk

The optic disk appears as a bright yellow region, similar to exudates. Therefore, we first detect the optic disk and prevent detecting false positive exudate lesions. Also, we try to detect the optic disk rim accurately since the estimated optic disk diameter allows to detect other retina structures, like the fovea center. For example, the fovea region can be located a number of optic disk diameters away from the optic disk center, in the temporal side of the optic disk [10]. Figure 2(a) depicts the input to our method, and Fig. 2(g) illustrates the output, that is, an image whose optic disk rim was automatically delimited. Thus, using this image we can find the optic disk center and the optic disk diameter accurately.

We developed a method that is adaptive to the local image intensity, for detecting the optic disk position and the optic disk rim [19]. Our method improves on other methods presented in the literature in terms of the accuracy of the optic disk rim detection, while it is not negatively influenced by the outgoing vessels confluence in the optic disk (a common difficulty in other methods [18]). In order to find the optic disk rim, we use the Watershed Transform from Markers [19]. Thus, we need to select internal and external markers to locate the optic disk boundaries (i.e. rim). In our method, we use several points situated inside the optic disk as internal markers. As external markers, we use several circles of constant diameter, centered at each previous selected internal marker. Then, using the Watershed Transform from Markers and the internal and external markers as parameters, several contour shapes are obtained. At last, we select the contour shape with the highest compactness and largest area to be the optic disk rim (see [19] for more details). In addition, in our work, the optic disk contour of each image has been labeled by four ophthalmologists as suggested in [11]. Figure 2(b)–(e) shows four ground truth images labeled by four ophthalmologists. Afterwards, the mean labeled contour was calculated, and then it was used as ground truth (see Fig. 2(f)). It shall be observed that color information in the eye fundus images contributes greatly to the identification of details in these images more accurately. According to our experts, color images are significantly better than grayscale images, and color information facilitates the image visual analysis.

3.2.2 Detecting the Fovea Center

We developed a new morphological approach for detecting the fovea center [20]. Our method relies on the existing spatial relationship between the optic disk and the macula to select a ROI (Region of Interest) in the green channel of the original color eye fundus image (see Fig. 3). Within this ROI, we detect fovea candidate regions using specific morphological filters. Afterwards, well known anatomical attributes of the fovea are used to validate its center location (e.g. the center of the darker candidate regions, located below the optic disk center, are selected). Figure 4 shows the main steps of our fovea center detection approach.

As illustrated in Fig. 5, our method identifies the fovea center as a pixel, and this method was validated on two publicly available databases of retinal images [20]. The fovea center detection accuracy is measured as the distance (in pixels) between the detected fovea center and the hand-labeled fovea center. In our experiments, we considered correct the detected fovea center that is distant no more than 50 pixels

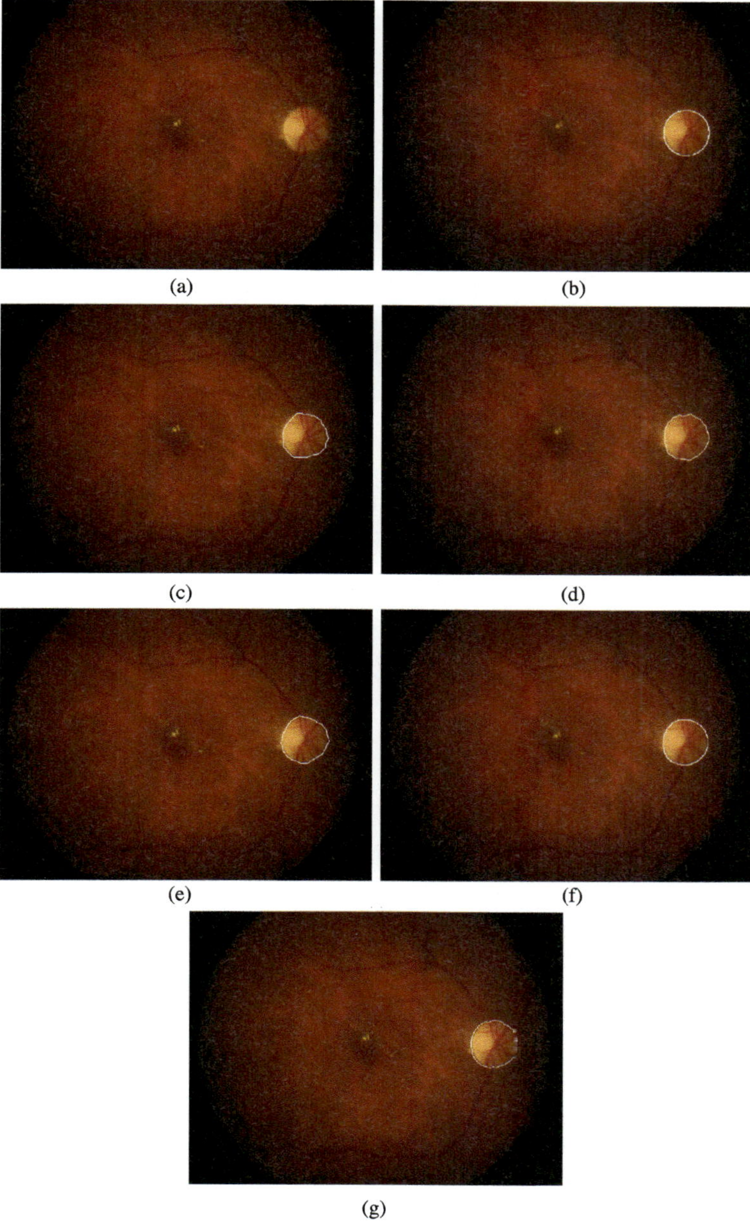

Fig. 2 (**a**) Color eye fundus image with exudates around the fovea center. (**b**)–(**e**) Shows four ground truth images labeled by four ophthalmologists (i.e. the optic disk were manually segmented by four ophthalmologists). (**f**) The mean labeled contour used as ground truth. (**g**) Detected optic disk rim on an image containing diabetic lesions

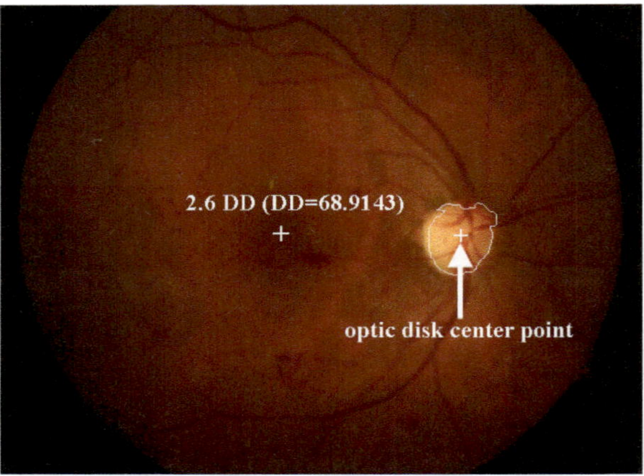

Fig. 3 Color eye fundus image with the optic disk center point and the fovea candidate region identified at 2.6 DD (disk diameter (DD), in this case, is equal to 68.9143 pixels)

from the ground truth (manually identified), as proposed by Niemeijer et al. [13]. Figure 5 shows the detected fovea center marked as a white dot superimposed on an original color eye fundus image of the DIARETDB1 database. Our method tends to be robust to artifacts near the fovea region, such as exudates, microaneurysms and microhemorrhages. The quantitative analysis using the Euclidean Distance and ground truth eye fundus images, indicate that our method tends to detect the fovea center more accurately than comparable approaches available in the literature. However, in the presence of large hemorrhages, our method may fail. The morphological filter used to remove the hemorrhages was able to remove small opaque lesions only, failing in the presence of large hemorrhages (see [20] for more details).

3.2.3 Detecting Exudate Lesions

The occurrence of exudate lesions near the central macular region may be the cause of severe visual loss. Therefore, the detection of exudate lesions and their proximity to the central macular region is essential for grading the Diabetic Macular Edema automatically. Our approach to detect exudates relies on mathematical morphology techniques and comprises three stages [21], namely: (a) preprocessing stage to adjust uneven illumination of the input image; (b) detection of exudates; and (c) post processing stage, to improve the exudates detection. All existing hard exudates on the images of DIARETDB1 database have been hand-labeled by experts, and then these hand-labeled images were taken as reference images (i.e. ground truth images) to validate our approach (see details in [21]).

Algorithm 1 describes the tree stages of our exudates lesion method. Lines 1 to 4 of Algorithm 1 describe the first stage. Lines 5 to 8 describe the second stage, and line 9 to 13 describe the third stage of our grading scheme. Briefly, $f1$ represents a background approximation of the L channel, and it is found by using alternating sequential filters of grayscale opening (i.e. γ) and grayscale closing (i.e. ϕ), where

Fig. 4 (**a**) A region of interest (ROI), of 160 × 160 pixels at 2.6 DD pixels of distance away from the optic disk center. This ROI was selected using the green channel of the original color eye fundus image. (**b**) ROI Image without signs of bright lesions (e.g. exudate lesions). (**c**) ROI image without small basins (e.g. microhemorrhages). (**d**) Fovea candidate regions. (**e**) Only candidate regions below the optic disk center point remain. (**f**) Selected region for the fovea. The centroid of this selected region is taken as the fovea center

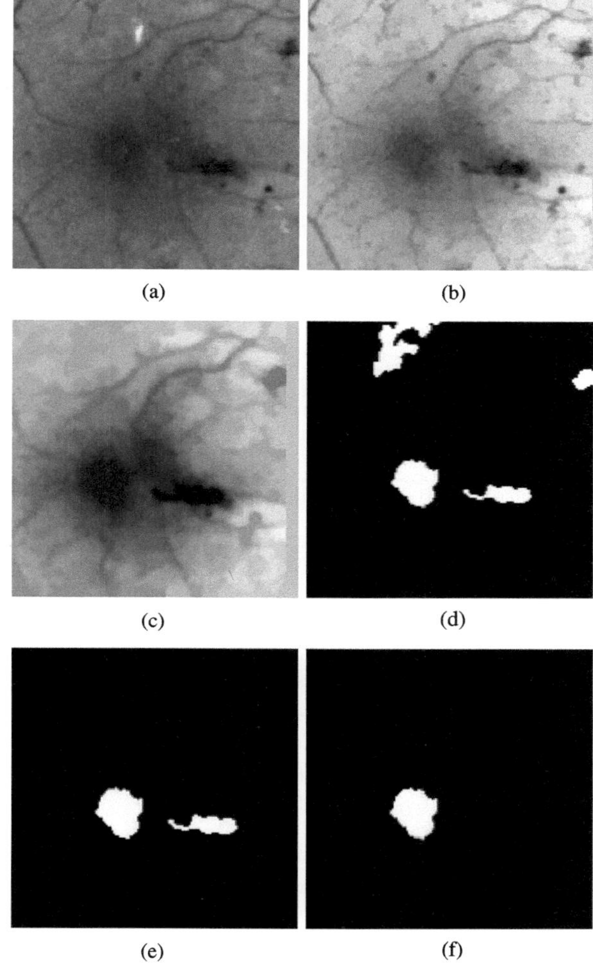

B is a fat, diamond-shaped, structuring element. We used in this work a diamond-shaped structuring element with a side of 80 pixels. This value represents the distance from the origin of this structuring element to the edge, and was obtained based on experiments. $f2$ represents an image without the smooth intensity variations of the background. The image $f3$ results from the removal of all connected basins from image $f2$ using the morphologic h-minima filter. $f4$ is an image that contains the set of all regional maxima, RMAX, of the image $f3$. Then, in order to detect the exudates candidate regions, an elementary dilation (i.e. δ) is performed on the image $f4$. Afterwards, we invert all the previously dilated regions to obtain the marker image $f5(x, y)$ (where $f_g(x, y)$ represents the green channel, of the original DIARETDB1 color image). B is a diamond-shaped structuring element, with a fixed radius 3. In the second stage, we find preliminary exudate lesion candidates by the following

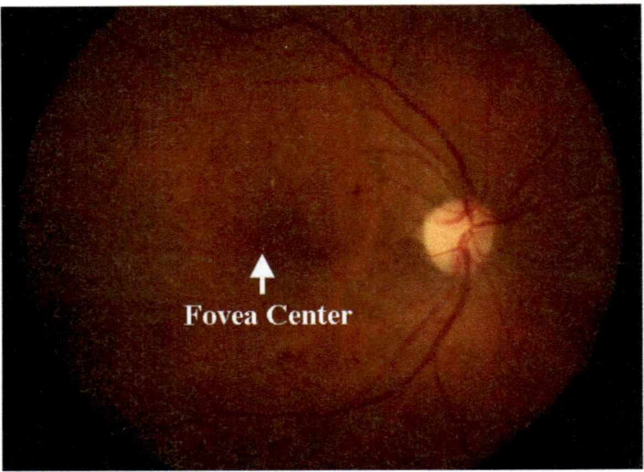

Fig. 5 Detected fovea center superimposed on the original color eye fundus image

---

Algorithm 1: Pseudo code to find exudate lesions using our tree steps approach [21]

Input: Color eye fundus image (RGB).
Output: Detected exudate lesions.

1 Convert the original RGB color image to L*u*v*;
2 Select the lightness scale, L as the input image;
3 $f1 = ((((L^* \; \gamma \; B) \; \phi \; B) \cdots \gamma \; nB) \; \phi \; nB)$;
4 $f2 = L^* - f1 + k$;
5 $f3 = hmin(f2) = \mathcal{R}^*_{f2}(f2 + h)$;
6 $f4 = RMAX(f3) = f3 + 1 - \mathcal{R}_{f3+1}(f3)$;
7 $f5(x, y) = \begin{cases} 0, & \text{if } \delta^{(B)}(f4(x, y)) = 1, \\ f_g(x, y), & \text{if } \delta^{(B)}(f4(x, y)) = 0; \end{cases}$
8 $f6(x, y) = \begin{cases} 0, & \text{if } (f_g - \mathcal{R}_{f_g}(f5)) \leq \lambda, \\ 1, & \text{if } (f_g - \mathcal{R}_{f_g}(f5)) > \lambda; \end{cases}$
9 $f7 = $ the binary image containing the vessel network;
10 $f8 = f6 - f7$;
11 $f9 = f_g + \gamma_{TH}(f_g) - \phi_{TH}(f_g)$;
12 $f10(x, y) = \begin{cases} 0, & \text{if } \delta^{(B)}(f8(x, y)) = 1, \\ f9(x, y), & \text{if } \delta^{(B)}(f8(x, y)) = 0; \end{cases}$
13 $f11(x, y) = \begin{cases} 0, & \text{if } (f9 - \mathcal{R}_{f9}(f10)) \leq \lambda, \\ 1, & \text{if } (f9 - \mathcal{R}_{f9}(f10)) > \lambda; \end{cases}$

---

steps. First, obtain a morphological reconstruction by dilation using the green channel f_g as a mask image and $f5$ as the marker image. Afterwards, we subtract the previously reconstructed image from the f_g image. Finally, we segment the exudate lesions using a thresholding algorithm, and a new binary image $f6$ is obtained. The vascular tree appears in the foreground of image $f7$, and this vascular tree is segmented using the method described in [19]. False positives (i.e. artifacts similar to exudates) appear in $f6$, and after refining these estimates by removing unlikely exudate estimates we obtain $f8$, which contains the (new) refined exudates candidate re-

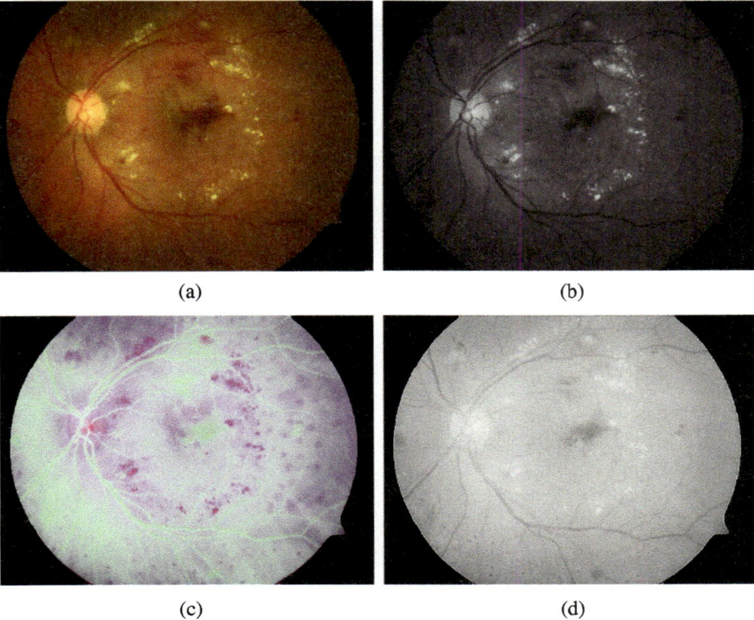

Fig. 6 (**a**) Original DIARETDB1 color eye fundus image. (**b**) Green channel of the original DIARETDB1 color eye fundus image. (**c**) L*u*v* color space of the original DIARETDB1 color eye fundus image. (**d**) L channel from L*u*v* color space

gions. *f9* in the line 11 of Algorithm 1 is an image morphologically enhanced, where γ_{TH} and ϕ_{TH} denote the morphological top-hat by opening and the morphological top-hat by closing operators, respectively. Moreover, we use a non-flat structuring element (i.e. B) with the shape of an ellipsoid to achieve our enhancement results. The radius of this structuring element was set to 12 pixels, and the reference height to gray level 50. Now, using the images *f8* and *f9*, we can find the last marker image *f10*, and the exudates are finally detected as shown in line 13 of Algorithm 1 ($\lambda = 5$ is all our experiments and B is a diamond-shaped structuring element, with a fixed radius 3). To implement the Algorithm 1, we used the MMORPH library [3]. See Ref. [21] for more details.

As described in Algorithm 1, was used L*u*v* color space to perform the first stages of our exudates lesion method. More precisely, we use the lightness L of the perceptually uniform L*u*v* color space in the first detection stage. It was observed that intensity fluctuations in the L channel are smaller than in the RGB channels [7]. Since we use global intensity information of the image, and such information appear to be less affected by illumination variation and noise in the L channel, we work with the L channel information to find the exudates. Figure 6(c) shows the L*u*v* color space of the original DIARETDB1 color eye fundus image (Fig. 6(a)). In addition, Fig. 6(d) illustrates the L channel from L*u*v* color space which presents less intensity fluctuations than the green channel (Fig. 6(b)) (see [21] for more details).

Table 2 Comparison of exudate detection methods (see [21] for more details)

Methods	Retinal Images with Hard-Exudates[a]			
	Average sensitivity	Average specificity	Average predictive value	Average misclassified proportion
Sopharak et al. [16]	43.48 %	99.31 %	25.48 %	0.68 %
Ravishankar et al. [14]	58.21 %	98.09 %	13.37 %	1.9 %
Walter et al. [18]	66.00 %	98.64 %	19.45 %	1.34 %
Our grading scheme method	72.21 %	98.97 %	21.65 %	1.0 %
Methods	Retinal Images without Hard-Exudates[b]			
	Average sensitivity	Average specificity	Average predictive value	Average misclassified proportion
Sopharak et al. [16]		99.28 %		0.71 %
Ravishankar et al. [14]		97.53 %		2.47 %
Walter et al. [18]		99.22 %		0.77 %
Our grading scheme method		99.40 %		0.6 %

[a]Comprises 47 images of the DIARETDB1 database

[b]Comprises 42 images of the DIARETDB1 database. The sensitivity and predictive value cannot be calculated because all TP (True Positives) and FN (False Negatives) values in color eye fundus images without exudates are equal to zero

Table 2 compares the grading scheme and other methods reported in the literature [21]. Our grading scheme achieved 72.21 % and 98.97 % of mean sensitivity and mean specificity, respectively, on the 47 images with hard-exudates. A comparison with other methods proposed in the literature is shown in Table 2, indicating that our method significantly improves on the results obtained by the other methods. Our method was also applied on retinal images without exudates, achieving a mean specificity of 99.40 % (i.e. the highest mean specificity value) and an average misclassified proportion of 0.6 % (i.e. the lowest misclassified proportion). However, as indicated in Table 2, the best average predictive and the lowest misclassified proportion were achieved by Sopharak et al. [16] on the retinal images with hard-exudates. Conversely, the method proposed by Sopharak et al. achieved the worst average sensitivity on the DIARETDB1. Let us clarify that sensitivity is the proportion (i.e. area in pixels) of true positives, TP, with respect to proportion of false negative, FN, pixels (i.e. $sensitivity = \frac{TP}{(TP+FN)}$). Specificity is the proportion of true negative, TN, pixels with respect to the proportion of false positive, FP, pixels (i.e. $specificity = \frac{TN}{(TN+FP)}$). However, as exudates occupy a small proportion of the whole image, specificity tends to be high, making it less meaningful. So, besides presenting specificity value, we also show the predictive values (i.e.

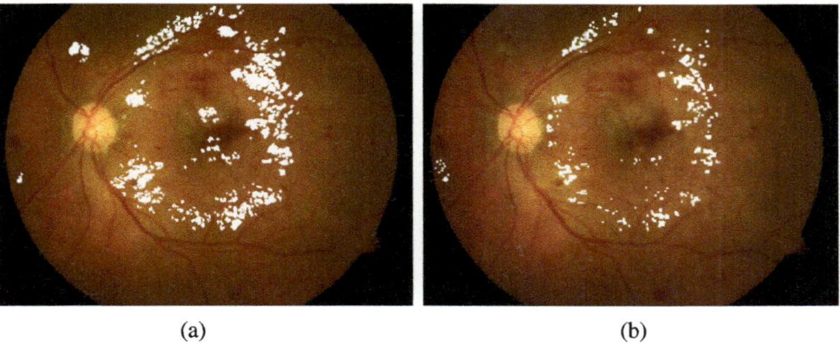

(a)   (b)

Fig. 7 (**a**) Detected exudates superimposed on an original DIARETDB1 color eye fundus image. (**b**) Ground truth image

predictive value $= \frac{TP}{(TP+FP)}$).[1] Additionally, we show the misclassified proportion, which is estimated as the proportion of pixels that are misclassified, or the proportion of false positives in the image (i.e. *misclassified proportion* $= \frac{FP}{(TP+FP+FN+TN)}$).

Figure 7 compares the result of our grading scheme for image #05 of the DIARETDB1 database with the ground truth image. Figure 7(a) shows the exudate lesions detected by our grading scheme (i.e. the detected exudates are depicted as bright spots). Figure 7(b) shows the ground truth image.

3.3 Lesion Signs Prescreening

In this section, we present the methods that locate the retinal sectors in an eye fundus image (see Sect. 3.3.1), and analyze the distribution of exudates in these retinal sectors (see Sect. 3.3.2).

3.3.1 Identification of Retinal Sectors

The detection of exudates is not sufficient for grading the Diabetic Macular Edema (DME) since the distribution of these exudates around the macula center also must be considered. For example, an eye fundus image containing more exudates may be associated to less harm to the patient visual condition than another eye fundus image containing less exudates, because in this last case the exudates may be closer to the macula center [10]. This exudates distribution is analyzed based on the retinal sectors, as shown in Fig. 8. The retinal image in sub-divided in 10 subfields (retinal sectors) [10, 16], namely: (1) Central; (2) Inner superior; (3) Inner temporal; (4) Inner inferior; (5) Inner nasal; (6) Outer superior; (7) Outer temporal; (8) Outer

---

[1]Predictive value is the probability that a certain pixel really is in an exudate region [18].

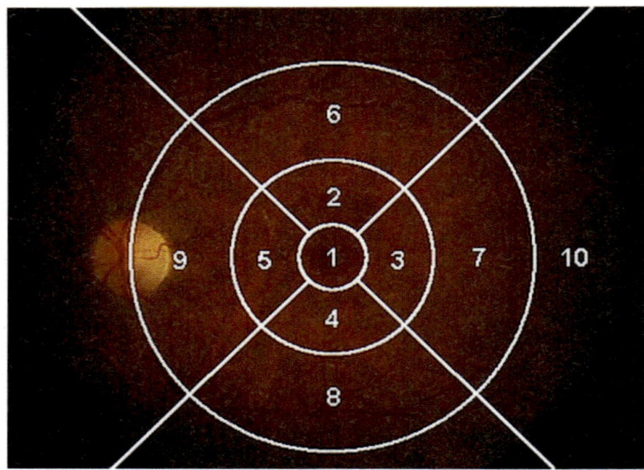

Fig. 8 Retinal sectors and its 10 subfields

inferior; (9) Outer nasal; (10) Far temporal subfield. These retinal sectors are centered at the fovea center, and the radii of the three fovea-centered circles are based on the optic disk diameter. The radii of the smaller, middle and outer fovea-centered circles are equal to $\frac{1}{3}$, 1 and 2 optic disk diameters, respectively [10].

3.3.2 Analyzing the Spatial Distribution of Exudate Lesions

The spatial distribution of exudates in an eye fundus image is analyzed based on the retinal sectors (subfields). Exudates inside the central circle (subfield 1) and inside of the inner circle (i.e. subfields 2–5), tend to affect more the patient visual acuity than the exudates inside (or beyond) the outer circle [10, 16]. For example, an eye fundus image showing several exudates located far from the macula center (e.g. inside or outside subfields 6–10) may indicate a less severe DME case, compared to another image showing fewer exudates near the macula center [10]. Figure 9(a) illustrates a color eye fundus image where most lesions are located near the macula center (inner superior and inner nasal subfield), indicating a severe DME case. On the other hand, Fig. 9(b) illustrates a color eye fundus image where most exudate lesions are located far from the macula center (outer temporal and far temporal subfield), indicating a mild DME case.

In our approach, exudates prescreening generates a table (namely, severity table) that describes the areas (in pixels) affected by exudates in the retina image subfields. Table 3 illustrates the severity table for the image in Fig. 9(a), indicating that exudates occur in 765 pixels in different subfields. In this example, there are exudate lesions in the central subfield and in the inner circle, indicating a severe DME case. The severity table may help grading DME cases, specially in the DME early stages when its potential impact on the patient visual acuity still can be reduced.

A DME case can be classified in terms of the severity table information as: (a) absent; (b) mild; (c) moderate; or (d) severe. Unfortunately, the *real world* probability density function (i.e. *pdf*) of the data in these classes is unknown. In complex data

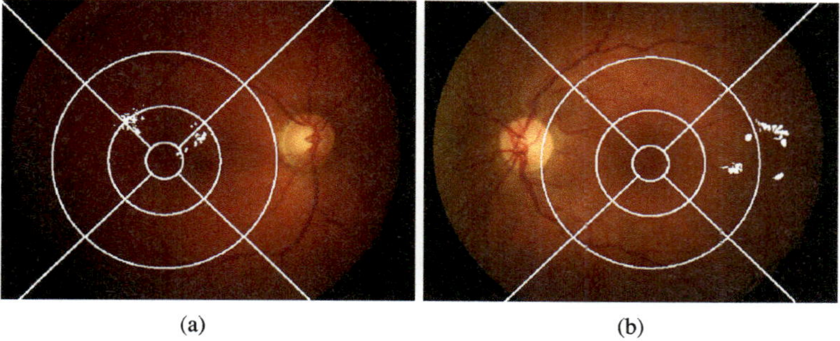

(a)   (b)

Fig. 9 Two images of the DIARETDB1 database with the exudates automatically identified and with the retinal sectors delimited. (**a**) Depict the image #03 of the DIARETDB1 database containing exudates in the central subfield, inner superior subfield, inner nasal subfield, inner temporal subfield, outer superior subfield and outer temporal subfield. (**b**) Depict the image #06 of DIARETDB1 database containing exudates far from the fovea, i.e. in the outer temporal subfield, far temporal subfield and in the outer superior subfield

Table 3 Location of exudates in Fig. 9(a), (b)

Region	Central	Inner			
		Superior	Nasal	Inferior	Temporal
Area	80	281	242	Absence	56
Region	Outer				Far Temporal
	Superior	Nasal	Inferior	Temporal	
Area	99	Absence	Absence	8	Absence
Total area	765 pixels				
Level	DME severe				

sets with intricate data relations (like in DME cases), large data sets are required to accurately estimate this *pdf*. Nevertheless, since each case corresponds to one patient, and the availability of patients in ophthalmology services is limited, the number of eye fundus images with DME signs often is too small for reliable *pdf* estimates. Therefore, in this work, we overcome this practical difficulty using the smoothed bootstrap approach,[2] where the statistical significance of the sample set is improved in each class by randomly re-sampling the original data to artificially produce another sample set, expanded maintaining a similar random structure. We approximate the unknown *pdf*s asymptotically, as the sample set is increased [4].

In order to determine the decision boundaries between the different classes (i.e. thresholds), the Classification and Regression Tree (CART) [1] method is used (the parameters are detailed in Sect. 4). The original data may be correlated, with adverse effects on the inter-class separability and the classification accuracy, and the

---

[2]Details of the smoothed bootstrap technique can be found in [4].

obtained data by bootstrapping the severity table data maintains a similar random structure. Therefore, CART was in fact used on a transformed data space, as detailed next.

Given a set of data samples A, the similarity matrix may be defined as a matrix S, where S_{ij} represents a similarity measure[3] between data samples $\mathbf{x_i}, \mathbf{x_j} \in A$. We apply a data clustering technique (i.e. CART) on the similarity matrix S spectrum to perform clustering in fewer dimensions, reducing the need for very large data sets to obtain data statistical significance. Also, the data tends to be less correlated and the inter-class separability often is improved in this spectral space. As proposed by Meila and Shi [12], we take the eigenvectors corresponding to the k' largest eigenvalues of the matrix $P = SD^{-1}$, where D is the diagonal matrix $D_{ii} = \sum_j S_{ij}$, and then cluster samples by their respective k' components in these eigenvectors. It is recommended that data is equally distributed among the 4 classes [12], therefore 1000 smoothed bootstrap data samples were generated for each DME severity class, summing up to 4000 data samples in total (all classes). These 4000 smoothed bootstrap data samples are clustered in the 4 DME severity classes by: (1) computing P from S, and its eigenvalues/vectors; (2) selecting the largest k' eigenvalues and their corresponding eigenvectors; (3) performing CART clustering into 4 classes by projecting the data samples $\mathbf{x}$ in the $k = k' - 1$ dimensional space defined by the rows of $[x_2, \ldots, x'_k]$. The inter-class boundaries are the thresholds found by CART.

4 Experimental Results

Our grading scheme was trained using smoothed bootstrap samples (see Sect. 3.3.2), and 35 DIARETDB1 color eye fundus images not in the training set were used for testing. The spectral space formed by $k = 3$ largest eigenvalues of the similarity matrix S produced the best results in our experiments, and was chosen to report our results. The 35 eye fundus images were screened by four retina experts and by our grading scheme, and the results are summarized in Table 4. Comparing with the mode of the experts classification (i.e. the class most voted by the experts in each case screened), our scheme graded incorrectly 2 DME cases (i.e. two false negatives were produced by our grading scheme, since in these two cases DME was misclassified as absent), obtaining an accuracy of 94.29 % in our experiments.

Confusion matrices were calculated for the four retina experts and for our grading scheme. Taking as a reference the mode of the DME grading done by the experts, the four experts obtained accuracies of 71.43 %, 94.29 %, 80 %, and 85.71 %, respectively, and their average accuracy was 82.86 %. Therefore, in our experiments our DME grading scheme obtained the same accuracy as Expert#2 (the most experienced among the experts), and a higher accuracy than the average of the four experts.

---

[3] $S_{ij} = e^{d(i,j)/\sigma}$, where $d(i, j)$ is the Euclidean distance between the data samples $\mathbf{x_i}$ and $\mathbf{x_j}$, and σ is a constant.

Table 4 Comparison of the DME severity level grading by our grading scheme and four retina experts, using 35 DIARETDB1 color eye fundus images with DME signs

	Severity level (manually assigned)					Severity level
	Expert#1	Expert#2	Expert#3	Expert#4	Mode	Our grading scheme
image#01	moderate	moderate	moderate	moderate	moderate	moderate
image#02	moderate	moderate	mild	moderate	moderate	moderate
image#03	moderate	moderate	mild	severe	moderate	moderate
image#04	severe	severe	severe	severe	severe	severe
image#05	severe	severe	severe	severe	severe	severe
image#06	mild	mild	absent	mild	mild	mild
image#07	severe	moderate	moderate	moderate	moderate	moderate
image#08	moderate	moderate	mild	moderate	moderate	moderate
image#09	moderate	moderate	moderate	severe	moderate	moderate
image#12	moderate	moderate	severe	moderate	moderate	moderate
image#13	moderate	moderate	moderate	moderate	moderate	moderate
image#14	moderate	moderate	moderate	moderate	moderate	moderate
image#15	moderate	moderate	severe	severe	severe	severe
image#16	moderate	severe	moderate	severe	severe	severe
image#17	mild	mild	mild	mild	mild	mild
image#18	moderate	mild	mild	mild	mild	mild
image#19	severe	severe	severe	severe	severe	severe
image#20	mild	mild	mild	moderate	mild	mild
image#21	absent	mild	mild	mild	mild	mild
image#24	moderate	moderate	moderate	moderate	moderate	moderate
image#25	moderate	moderate	severe	severe	severe	severe
image#26	mild	mild	mild	mild	mild	mild
image#35	mild	moderate	moderate	moderate	moderate	absent
image#38	mild	moderate	moderate	moderate	moderate	moderate
image#49	absent	absent	absent	absent	absent	absent
image#50	absent	absent	absent	absent	absent	absent
image#51	absent	absent	absent	absent	absent	absent
image#53	mild	moderate	moderate	severe	moderate	moderate
image#58	absent	absent	absent	absent	absent	absent
image#60	absent	absent	absent	absent	absent	absent
image#62	absent	absent	absent	absent	absent	absent
image#66	moderate	moderate	mild	moderate	moderate	moderate
image#75	absent	absent	absent	absent	absent	absent
image#84	moderate	moderate	moderate	severe	moderate	absent
image#86	moderate	absent	absent	absent	absent	absent
Accuracy	71.43 %	94.29 %	80 %	85.71 %		94.29 %

5 Conclusions and Future Trends

The growing amount of medical information (e.g. the vast amount of existing medical imaging modalities) requires the use of computer-aided diagnosis systems. For instance, when the computer-aided diagnosis systems are used in clinical practice, the patient care can be more efficient. Moreover, the same computer-aided system can be used in the training of future medical specialists. However, it is important to note that the automatic diagnostic methods may fail, and therefore can not be used for clinical practice in an isolated way. These methods should be seen as a decision support system and their use should always be assisted by an expert. In this chapter, we present a scheme for detecting and grading Diabetic Macular Edema (DME) signs in color eye fundus images. Our DME grading scheme detects retina structures and lesion signs, and then classifies the lesions signs spatial distribution in the retina image subfields. The output of our DME grading scheme is a severity table and an estimated severity level, which may help in the objective evaluation of the potential impact of DME on the patient visual acuity. Our preliminary experimental results are promising, since our grading scheme potentially can grade automatically DME cases with a performance similar to an expert. Future work will concentrate on an extensive clinical evaluation of our grading scheme, and on investigating the application of the proposed DME grading scheme in telemedicine.

References

1. Alpaydin E (2004) Introduction to machine learning. Adaptive computation and machine learning. The MIT Press, Cambridge
2. Ciulla TA, Amador AG, Zinman B (2003) Diabetic retinopathy and diabetic macular edema. Diabetes Care 26(9):2653–2664
3. Dougherty ER, Lotufo RA (2003) Hands-on morphological image processing. SPIE publications, vol TT59
4. Franke J, Halim S (2007) Wild bootstrap tests. IEEE Signal Process Mag 24(4):31–37
5. Goh KG, Hsu W, Lee ML, Wang H (2001) ADRIS: an automatic diabetic retinal image screening system. In: Medical data mining and knowledge discovery. Springer, Berlin, pp 181–210
6. Hayashi JI, Kunieda T, Cole J, Soga R, Hatanaka Y, Lu M, Hara T, Fujita H (2001) A development of computer-aided diagnosis system using fundus images. In: Proceedings of the seventh international conference on virtual systems and multimedia (VSMM'01). IEEE Computer Society, Los Alamitos
7. Jähne B, Haußecker H, Geißler P (1999) Handbook of computer vision and applications: signal processing and pattern recognition, vol 2. Academic Press, New York
8. Kauppi T, Kalesnykiene V, Kämäräinen JK, Lensu L, Sorri I, Raninen A, Voutilainen R, Uusitalo H, Kälviäinen H, Pietilä J (2007) DIARETDB1 diabetic retinopathy database and evaluation protocol. In: Medical image understanding and analysis (MIUA), pp 61–65
9. Lalonde M, Laliberté F, Gagnon L (2004) RetsoftPlus: a tool for retinal image analysis. In: Proceedings of the 17th IEEE symposium on computer-based medical systems (CBMS'04). IEEE, New York, pp 542–547
10. Li H, Chutatape O (2004) Automated feature extraction in color retinal images by a model based approach. IEEE Trans Biomed Eng 51(2):246–254
11. Lowell J, Hunter A, Steel D, Basu A, Ryder R, Fletcher E, Kennedy L (2004) Optic nerve head segmentation. IEEE Trans Med Imaging 23(2):256–264

12. Meila M, Shi J (2001) A random walks view of spectral segmentation. International conference on AI and statistics (AISTAT)
13. Niemeijer M, Abràmoff MD, Ginneken BV (2007) Segmentation of the optic disc, macula and vascular arch in fundus photographs. IEEE Trans Med Imaging 26:116–127
14. Ravishankar S, Jain A, Mittal A (2009) Automated feature extraction for early detection of diabetic retinopathy in fundus images. In: IEEE conference on computer vision and pattern recognition (CVPR). IEEE, Miami
15. Simandjuntak RA, Suksmono AB, Mengko TLR, Sovani I (2005) Development of computer-aided diagnosis system for early diabetic retinopathy based on micro aneurysms detection from retinal images. In: Proceedings of 7th international workshop on enterprise networking and computing in healthcare industry, HEALTHCOM 2005. IEEE, New York, pp 364–367
16. Sopharak A, Uyyanonvara B, Barmanb S, Williamson TH (2008) Automatic detection of diabetic retinopathy exudates from non-dilated retinal images using mathematical morphology methods. Comput Med Imaging Graph 32:720–727
17. Tobin KW, Chaum E, Govindasamy VP, Karnowski TP (2007) Detection of anatomic structures in human retinal imagery. IEEE Trans Med Imaging 26(12):1729–1739
18. Walter T, Klein JC, Massin P, Erginay A (2002) A contribution of image processing to the diagnosis of diabetic retinopathy—detection of exudates in color fundus images of the human retina. Trans Med Imaging 21(10):1236–1243
19. Welfer D, Scharcanski J, Kitamura CM, Pizzol MMD, Ludwig LWB, Marinho DR (2010) Segmentation of the optic disk in color eye fundus images using an adaptive morphological approach. Comput Biol Med 40(2):124–137
20. Welfer D, Scharcanski J, Marinho DR (2009) A morphological approach for the fovea location in color fundus images. In: International conference on information technology and communications in health. ITCH. Laurel point Inn, Victoria
21. Welfer D, Scharcanski J, Marinho DR (2010) A morphologic three-stage approach for detecting exudates in color eye fundus images. In: 25th symposium on applied computing, ACM SAC'10. ACM, Sierre
22. World Health Organization (2005) Prevention of blindness from diabetes mellitus: report of a WHO consultation in Geneva, Switzerland. Tech rep
23. Yen GG, Leong WF (2008) A sorting system for hierarchical grading of diabetic fundus images: a preliminary study. Trans Inf Technol Biomed 12(1):118–130

Colour Image Analysis of Wireless Capsule Endoscopy Video: A Review

Mark Fisher and Michal Mackiewicz

Abstract Wireless capsule endoscopy (CE) has been available since 2001 and is now established as one of the principal approaches used to examine the small bowel, with a range of devices available from four manufacturers. But although its use is widespread the reading of CE videos remains an arduous and time consuming exercise for gastroenterologists because relevant frames which are of interest to the physician constitute only about 1 % of the video. CE exam viewing times vary from 40–90 minutes, depending on the clinician's experience, the complexity of the case and the small bowel transit time. Colour image analysis has been applied by manufacturers to speed up this process, for example, Given Imaging's *Rapid Reader* Software includes a suspected blood indicator (SBI) designed to detect bleeding in the video. However, some evaluations of this tool reported concerns with regard to its specificity and sensitivity and so it does not free the specialist from reviewing the entire footage and can only be used as a fast screening aid. Over the past decade a number of papers have proposed a range of colour image processing and computer vision applications to assist the gastroenterologist in the analysis of CE video. These techniques can be divided into three categories, the first considers the topographic segmentation of CE video into meaningful parts such as mouth, oesophagus, stomach, small intestine, and colon. The second involves the detection of clinically significant video events (both abnormal and normal) and the third attempts to adaptively adjust the video viewing speed. This chapter reviews this research focusing particularly on the role of colour and texture descriptors and concludes by suggesting possible future directions for CE analysis.

M. Fisher (✉) · M. Mackiewicz
School of Computing Sciences, University of East Anglia, Norwich Research Park, Norwich, NR4 7TJ, UK
e-mail: Mark.Fisher@uea.ac.uk

M. Mackiewicz
e-mail: M.Mackiewicz@uea.ac.uk

M.E. Celebi, G. Schaefer (eds.), *Color Medical Image Analysis*,
Lecture Notes in Computational Vision and Biomechanics 6,
DOI 10.1007/978-94-007-5389-1_7, © Springer Science+Business Media Dordrecht 2013

1 Introduction

Wireless Capsule Endoscopy (CE) is a non-invasive clinical procedure allowing the entire Gastrointestinal (GI) tract to be examined using a small encapsulated CMOS camera. The development of this system was heralded in 2000 [1] and the first commercial system was available from Given Imaging Ltd. following FDA (American Food and Drug Administration) clearance in August 2001. The system, initially marketed as *M2A* but later rebranded *PillCam SB* (SB denoting Small Bowel), consists of a small (11 mm × 26 mm) capsule, an associated data-recorder belt and application software. The disposable capsule is swallowed and propelled through the GI tract by peristalsis before being expelled naturally. A transparent optical dome at one end of the capsule contains an array of six white light emitting diodes which surround a camera designed to capture two (256 × 256) colour images a second. The images are compressed by JPEG and transmitted using radiotelemetry to the data recorder which is worn by the patient on a belt. Analysis of the RF signal received by an array of aerials fixed to the patient's body allows the position of the capsule to be determined and its trajectory to be logged. Two silver-oxide batteries located at the other end of the capsule enable the camera to operate for about 8 hours, after such time the belt is removed for analysis. A software application called *Rapid Reader* allows the stored data (approximately 50,000 images) to be downloaded to a PC workstation for analysis. The clinical procedure is simple. The patient is advised to fast overnight and in some cases a drug which prepares the bowel and reduces GI transit time is administered. On the following morning, antennas are attached to the patient and connected to the data recorder, which is worn on a belt. The physician removes the capsule from its holder and performs a visual check to confirm it is operational before it is ingested by the patient. Once the capsule has been swallowed the patient is free to undertake normal tasks (subject to certain limitations), returning to hospital after a period of 8 hours has elapsed.

In 2004 Given Imaging launched a second product called *PillCam ESO*, incorporating two CMOS cameras (one positioned at each end of the capsule) operating at a higher frame rate designed to target oesophageal disease. *PillCam COLON*, launched in 2006, represents another specialization of the concept, optimized for colon examinations. PillCam COLON also employs two cameras but after activation the capsule enters a sleep mode for two hours (allowing it to reach the colon) before resuming image transmission. In 2005 Olympus launched a system called *EndoCapsule* with similar functionality to *PillCam SB*. *EndoCapsule* uses a CCD camera system equipped with automatic brightness control (ABC) to provide automatic illumination adjustment designed to deliver higher resolution images of consistent quality. A unique feature of *EndoCapsule* is a real-time viewer which allows the clinician to observe images as they are captured in addition to reviewing the video using the more usual off-line analysis tool (*EndoView*). Given responded in 2007 by launching *PillCam SB 2* a second-generation product with a superior specification and additional features designed to improve workflow. Subsequent second generation versions denoted *PillCam ESO 2* and *PillCam COLON 2* followed. Since 2007, capsules called *MicroCam* developed by IntroMedic and a Chinese competitor called *OMOM* (jinshangroup.com) have become available. The stream of images

Fig. 1 *Rapid Reader* v4
(Given Imaging)

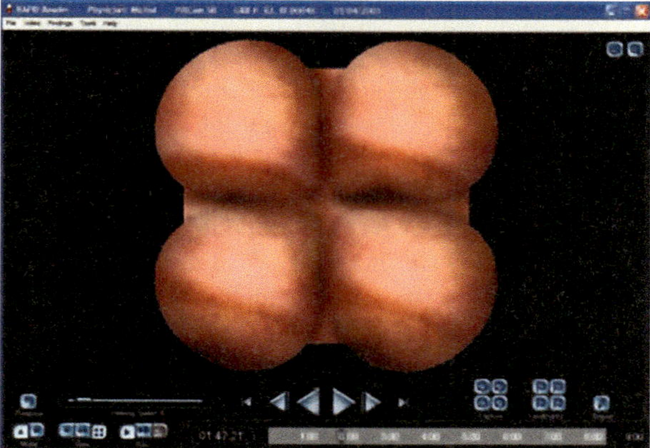

Fig. 2 *EndoView* (Olympus)

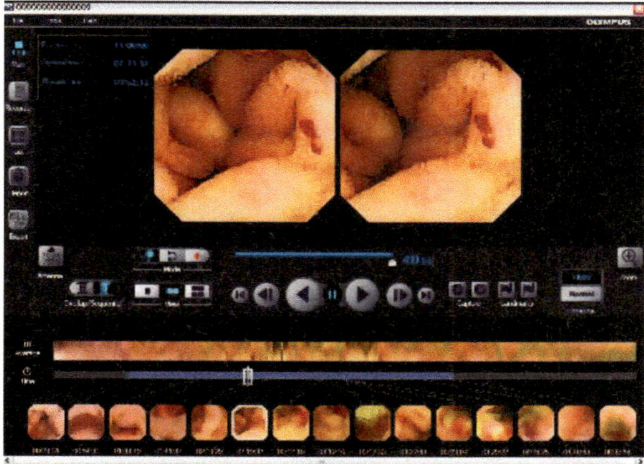

captured by the data recorder are presented as a video (typically 30 mins) and analyzed by a trained clinician using application software supplied by the manufacturer (e.g. Figs. 1 and 2).

The analysis software packages provided by different manufacturers comprise tools designed to improve the workflow and reduce the time spent on the analysis task (typically somewhere between 45–90 mins). In [2], the authors comment that with the expected reduction in capsule prices, the time needed by a clinician to analyse the exam may soon become the most expensive part of the procedure. Thus, a reduction of this time would be a major benefit, provided the quality of the diagnostic report was not reduced. The existing systems have user-friendly viewing interfaces, but with few exceptions lack automated tools that would highlight places of interest. Such tools could not only shorten the exam viewing time, but also improve the quality of patient's diagnosis by drawing attention to possible pathology, which could have been missed by the clinician among many thousands of normal frames. Incidentally, the manufacturers of the capsule try to reduce the video viewing time using additional viewing controls e.g. double and quad views in the *Rapid Reader* and *EndoView* software packages.

It is here where the computer vision can make a significant impact on the utility of CE. Ultimately, we would want the computer to take over from the clinician in stating the diagnosis allowing for a much cheaper screening technique. While this is still a very remote possibility, the development of computer vision methods for CE already allows or will soon allow for a significant aid in clinician's diagnosis. From segmenting CE video sequence into meaningful anatomical parts to detecting bleeding and other possible pathologies, computer vision methods have matured since the introduction of the first capsule a decade ago. The biggest challenge these algorithms face is to prove themselves that they can be trusted in practice i.e. perform the designated task at least as accurately as clinicians and hence allow for their wider adoption in clinical tools relieving clinicians from the burden of time consuming analysis. The ultimate bottom line measure here is the false negative ratio as for example for the pathological video event detection task, the exam evaluated as *normal* could skip manual inspection streamlining the population screening process.

The rest of this chapter reviews the computer vision research focusing particularly on the role of colour and texture descriptors and concludes by suggesting possible future directions for CE analysis. The main subjects of research are topographic video segmentation and filtering of non-informative frames, designed to provide a focus of attention, and classifiers for bleeding and abnormality detection. The following sections examine research in these areas, focusing in particular on the way that colour information is used in these tasks.

1.1 Feature Extraction

The distribution of colours in an image provides a useful cue for image indexing and object recognition. The colour distribution histogram is the most commonly used method of representing image colour information [3]. It is relatively invariant to image scale changes, translation and rotation about the viewing axis, and partial occlusion. Colour is an effective cue in CE image analysis and a salient feature of many proposed algorithms. Visually, the colour of the mouth is unsaturated, the stomach pinkish; the small intestine pinkish to yellowish; and the colon also pinkish to yellowish but often occluded by varying amounts of yellowish to greenish colour caused by faecal contamination. Moreover, different pathologies have their own distinct colour signatures. For example, ulcerations often contain yellowish and white colours surrounded by the overly reddish hues suggesting inflammation or bleeding.

CE video frames are stored as RGB triplets but very few researchers choose to analyse the data in this form. Fox [4], Bourbakis et al. [5] and Hwang et al. [6] are amongst a minority who extract colour features directly from RGB colour space. The authors claim their blood classifier appears to outperform the SBI tool provided by Given Imaging. Building on the work of Swain and Ballard [3], Berens [7] explored the scalability of colour indexing and extended their work by investigating

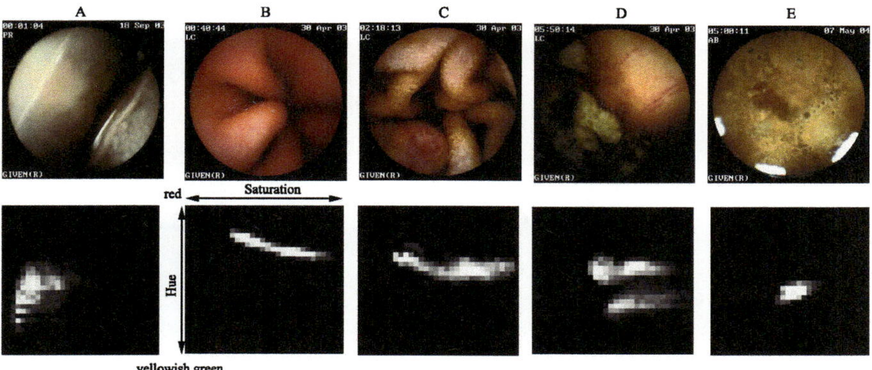

Fig. 3 CE images acquired from (**A**) Mouth, (**B**) Stomach, (**C**) Small Intestine, (**D**) partially occluded Colon and (**E**) completely occluded Colon; and below their respective equalized HS histograms. A visible shift in hue (vertical axis of the histogram) between the respective histograms is clearly visible. From [13]

the choice of colour space, coding of color histograms and techniques to provide invariance to illumination. Experiments undertaken by Berens [8, 9] showed that RGB colour space is not the best choice for image classification and that other perceptually relevant colour spaces such as HSI (Hue, Saturation, Intensity) produced better classification results. Consequently, Mackiewicz, working with Berens and Fisher, [10–13] also use HSI colour space, but due to the range of intensity variation in CE images, arising as the distance between the capsule and the intestine surface constantly varies, they ignore the intensity channel and favour HS histograms. The range of colour present in CE images is relatively small, mapping to a region covering just around 20 % of the possible HS colour space, so the histograms are equalized within this subset of red to yellowish-green colours. Figure 3 shows typical CE images acquired from the mouth, stomach, intestine and colon regions, and their respective HS histograms. It can be seen that the colour distribution of the stomach is slightly shifted towards red, compared to that within the intestine. It is also clear that the colour distribution of the colon tissue is highly similar to that of the small intestine, when it is free of faecal contamination. However, colon images are generally obscured by the presence of faecal contamination which has a distinct hue-saturation signature.

Texture features can play an important role, particularly in topographic video segmentation of CE video (Sect. 2). The most prominent texture pattern that distinguishes different organs are small finger-like projections called villi (responsible for food absorption), visible in Fig. 3C. These are present in the small intestine, but not in the neighbouring regions of stomach and colon. Mackiewicz et al. analyse texture by employing a 3D Local Binary Pattern (LBP) operator introduced by Connah and Finlayson [14] which extends the concept originally conceived by Mäenpää and Pietikäinen [15–17] who calculated 1D LBP histograms for the three colour channels independently. Because CE images are often obscured (to a varying degree) by

Fig. 4 Grid of 28 sub-image
regions. From [13]

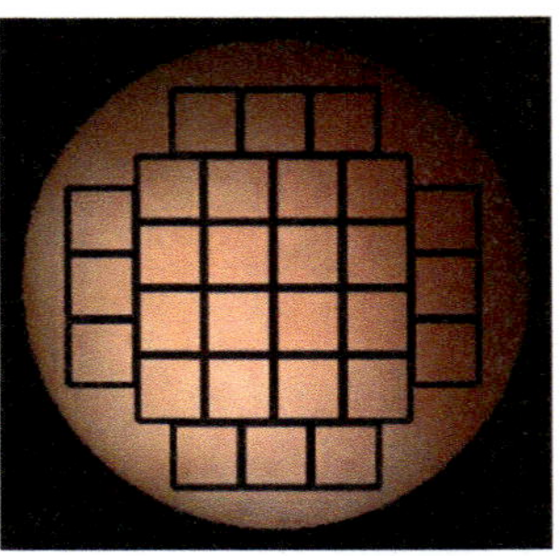

strong shadows, or by air bubbles and other artifacts such as mucus, bile, faeces, food etc. histograms built using the entire image will contain any visual contamination present in the image. To address this problem, some researchers extract only those parts of the image which contain only non-occluded tissue. In this respect, Mackiewicz divides each CE image frame into a grid of 28 sub-image regions arranged to cover most of the image area as shown in Fig. 4 and discards those regions which do not meet certain conditions.

The criteria are based on testing five parameters: Mean Intensity, Saturation, Hue, and Standard Deviation of Intensity and Hue against similar values derived from visually clear images of gastrointestinal tissue. The remaining sub-images form a so-called *sub-image region* (SubIR) that is used by the feature extraction process described previously. Figure 5 shows eight typical images acquired in the stomach and intestine showing only those sub-images selected by the procedure described above.

Another key result of Berens's work was that transform coding could be used to efficiently represent colour histograms without degrading their indexing performance [8, 18]. Mackiewicz applies this idea to colour histograms derived from CE images using both DCT and PCA transforms in a two stage algorithm to reduce the colour feature vector to just 8 values. Figure 6 shows the first three principal components calculated using the Hybrid Transform (DCT followed by PCA) from 1000 HS histograms extracted from one CE video. Each dot on the graph represents one histogram.

Jeongkyu Lee et al. [19] also address the problem of event boundary detection in CE arguing that there is compelling evidence to suggest HSI provides strong features that are highly correlated with topographic segments of the GI tract. Li et al. [20–22] also adopt the HSI colour space but in a similar approach to Mackiewicz they only use the HS components, summarizing this feature as a so called *chromaticity moment*. Coimbra et al. [23–27] favour colour and texture descriptors drawn from the MPEG-7 standard [28] and have evaluated these for detecting a variety of events in CE video. In [25] they conclude that the MPEG-7 *Scalable Colour* (SC) and *Homogeneous Texture* (HT) descriptors are the most adequate for the task of event detection. The SC descriptor is derived from the colour histogram defined in the HSI color space with fixed color space quantization of 16 bins. For compression, this information is encoded using the Haar transform, allowing scalable representa-

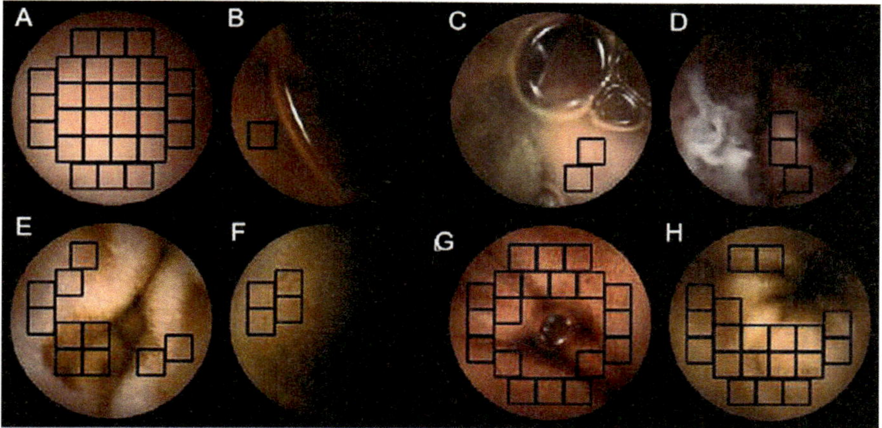

Fig. 5 CE images showing selected SubIRs. **A–D** Stomach; **E–H** Intestine. From [13]

Fig. 6 Three first principal components representing compressed histograms extracted from four different video regions. From [13]

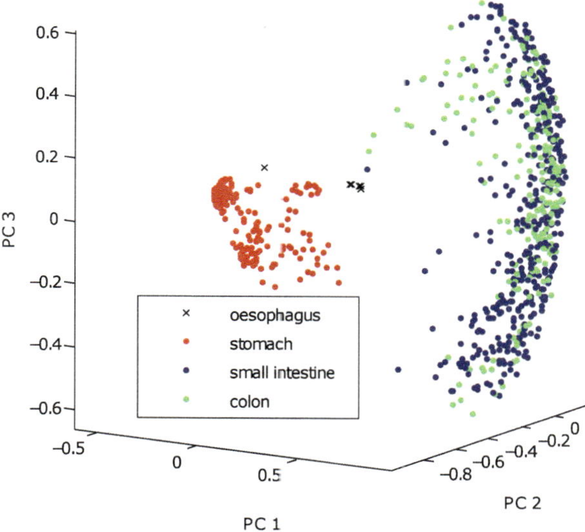

tion of the description and complexity scalability of feature extraction and matching procedures [29]. The HT descriptor encodes a precise statistical distribution of the image texture as a vector of 62 integers coming from the Gabor filter response of 30 frequency channels quantized in 30° radial segments in 5 octave bands [30]. Duda et al. [31, 32] also test MPEG-7 descriptors for CE image discrimination and conclude that the HT descriptor is the most reliable and the colour descriptors all performed similarly. They also selected HT and SC descriptors as features. In their work, Vilarino et al. [33–35] also surveyed a range of image descriptors and concluded that intensity, color and texture are the most relevant visual cues when processing endoscopic videos. However, since their focus is intestinal contractions they pursue a sequence-based rather than a frame-based approach, focusing on variations in image intensity.

All researchers use colour features as inputs, sometimes combined with other cues derived from motion, to classify single images and image sequences drawn from CE video. Applications fall broadly into three areas. Topographic video segmentation, the detection of clinically significant abnormalities, and attempts to control the speed at which frames are delivered to the viewer. These are reviewed in Sects. 2, 3 and 4.

2 Topographic Video Detection

The GI tract comprises mouth, oesophagus, stomach and duodenum (upper GI tract), the jejunum, ileum, colon and rectum. Typically the capsule takes a few seconds to pass through the oesophagus before reaching the esogastric junction and entering the stomach. The capsule remains in the stomach typically 15 minutes but this period might be extended to several hours before it passes through the pylorus (a valve between the stomach and the small intestine). The capsule takes about four hours to transit the small intestine before entering the colon. Three key landmarks are the esogastric junction (between oesophagus and stomach), pylorus (between stomach and small intestine), and ileocaecal valve (between small intestine and colon). Annotating the esogastric junction is quite easy as the features inside the mouth, oesophagus and stomach are quite different. Locating the pylorus in the video can be difficult and time consuming, even for those experienced in this task, as the stomach tissue near the pyloric valve and that of the small intestine are visually similar. The ileocaecal valve which marks the entry to the colon is even more difficult to locate as the tissue is often obscured by faecal material.

Topographic video segmentation considers the problem of segmenting the capsule video into meaningful parts such as mouth, oesophagus, small intestine and colon. Researchers have observed that the choice of the right features is probably the most important issue in this segmentation task and most support the view that image texture is an important cue. Mackiewicz and Coimbra classify single images based on information recovered from colour and texture descriptors (combined with a motion descriptor) and use these results to classify image features into the previously mentioned anatomical classes. Work by both Coimbra and Mackiewicz concludes that using a Support Vector Classifier rather than a Bayesian approach improves the results, which can then be used within a navigation tool and to estimate the capsule Gastric and Intestinal Transit Times, which are important factors in diagnosing certain medical conditions.

Mackiewicz investigates a number of recognition algorithms including various linear and non-linear classifiers: Multivariate Gaussian, kNN and Support Vector Classifier (SVC) to perform the actual video segmentation, i.e. label the transition points between anatomical regions. He performs a number of experiments to test his topographic segmentation approach using a data set comprising 76 annotated

CE videos provided by clinical collaborators at the Norfolk and Norwich University Hospital. The videos were annotated by an experienced clinician and segmented into meaningful parts: Entrance, Stomach, Intestine and Colon. The input feature set comprised both colour features derived from both whole images and subIRs. Single images are classified as Entrance/Stomach, Stomach/Intestine and Intestine/Colon. In these experiments the HS histograms were quantized into $32 \times 32 = 1024$ bins and LBP histograms were built using 8 sampling points to provide 7 unique patterns, $21(3 \times 7)$ bins for the independent 1D histogram and $343(7^3)$ for the joint 3D histogram.

It is worth noting that the choice of anatomical regions to be segmented varied between researchers. The most popular set was mouth/entrance; oesophagus; stomach; small intestine and colon. However, Duda et al. attempted to classify the CE images from only the upper part of the GI tract into a larger number of distinctive regions. They chose six anatomical regions: (A) oesophagus, (B) cardia, (C) fundus, (D) corpus of the stomach, (E) pylorus and (F) duodenal cap. They used Neural Networks as the image feature classifiers. The authors reported only the classification results and did not attempt to segment the actual videos. Lee et al. chose yet another set of anatomical regions namely: oesophagus; stomach; duodenum and jejunum; ileum; and colon. The idea for their algorithm is based on the fact that each digestive organ has different patterns of intestinal contractions. The analysis of the frequency functions associated to these patterns leads to the event boundaries which indicate either entrance to the consecutive organ or unusual events in the same organ, such as intestinal juices, bleeding, ulceration, and unusual capsule movements. These events can then be classified and if necessary merged into higher level events that represent digestive organs leading to a tree-like representation of the capsule endoscopy topography. The authors report that the performance on ileum and colon is worse than on the upper digestive organs which confirms the earlier findings regarding difficulties with locating the entrance to the colon reported by Mackiewicz and Coimbra.

Some researchers have produced clinical demonstrator systems by combining their classifiers within a search framework that allows the user to search and navigate within and between topographic regions. Both Coimbra and Mackiewicz have found a Hidden Markov Model (HMM) to be the best strategy for this purpose.

3 Detection of Clinically Significant Events

Another important research area involves the detection of clinically significant video events (both abnormal and normal). Examples include physical abnormality (e.g. ulceration, polyp, cancer), intestinal fluids, intestinal contractions and capsule retention. This category also includes bleeding, an area which has received considerable focus in the literature and one that has been addressed by the manufacturers in their proprietary software packages.

Blood detection is a focus for much of CE research, perhaps motivated by early reports that questioned the performance of the SBI shipped with *PillCam SB*.

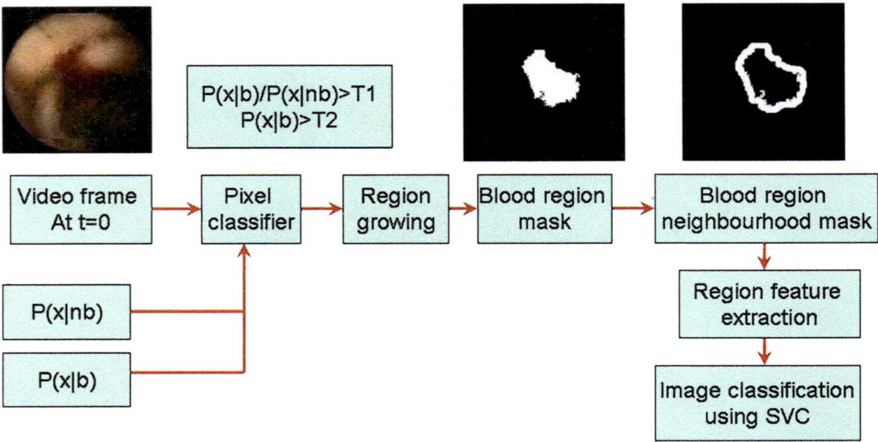

Fig. 7 Bleeding detection system flow chart. From [13]

In [4, 6], the authors propose a new algorithm that they claim can detect bleeding areas in the capsule videos. The algorithm uses Expectation Maximization (EM) clustering and Bayesian Information Criterion (BIC). The authors manually segmented around 200 images into blood and non-blood regions. Then, they selected 16,000 bleeding and 45,000 non-bleeding pixels and modelled the colour distribution of these regions using Gaussian mixtures in RGB colour space. A Bayesian decision rule was used. The algorithm chooses those pixels x to be bleeding candidates for which conditional probability $p(x—bleeding)$ of a pixel x given by bleeding pixels is significantly larger than conditional probability $p(x—non-bleeding)$ of a pixel x given by non-bleeding pixels; and also it is larger than a certain predefined threshold. In the final step of the algorithm, the areas of bleeding regions are calculated and all segmented regions containing less than 1,000 pixels are rejected. To test the results of bleeding detection, the authors selected 15,222 capsule images of which 1,731 contained blood from three different videos. On this test set, the reported specificity and sensitivity were 98,10 % and 92,55 % respectively.

Contrary to [4, 6], who use parametric bleeding colour distribution models, Mackiewicz chooses a different method using the similar feature set as described in the previous section [36]. A simplified flowchart of the bleeding detection system is shown in Fig. 7. First, each pixel is classified as bleeding or non-bleeding using a HSI model. Then, a region growing operation merges candidate pixels into regions of at least 250 pixels. If a blood region is detected, associated colour and texture features are extracted. These features are also extracted from the region surrounding the suspicious region. Then, after searching for specular highlights in order to check if the frame contains air bubbles, these features are used to identify the frame as containing suspicious regions. The images are classified using a Support Vector Classifier into three classes: Bleeding, Lesion/Abnormality or Normal, reporting figures of 97 %, 92 % and 92 % respectively using on ten-fold cross validation with a database comprising 84 full-length CE videos.

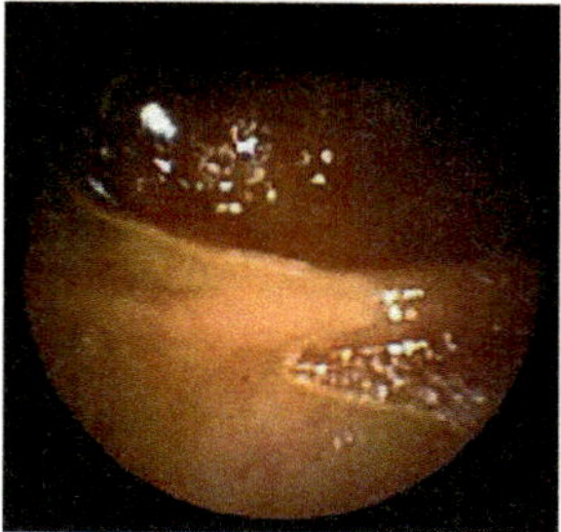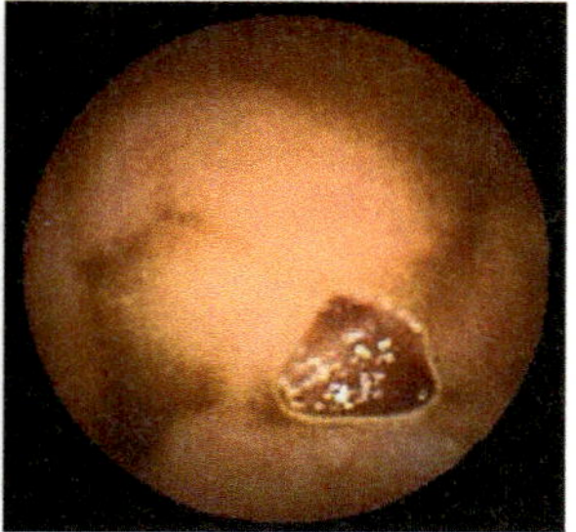

Fig. 8 Two images containing air bubbles with specular highlights. From [13]

Another idea for aiding capsule endoscopy video review involves removing non-informative frames from the video sequence. Early detection of such regions is highly beneficial since they can be removed from the sequence, before it is presented to the clinician, resulting in a shortening of the reviewing time. Intestinal fluids are one type of non-informative content. They appear as yellowish to brownish semi-opaque turbid liquids often containing air-bubbles as well as other artifacts (Fig. 8). Removal of such frames was first proposed by [34] who presented an algorithm which detects areas in the WCE video comprising images completely obscured by intestinal fluids. The authors observe that the most relevant feature of the intestinal fluids is the presence of small bubbles of different sizes and quasi-circular shapes. Their algorithm is based on texture analysis performed using Gabor filter banks. In order to construct a filter bank, the authors used four different directions oriented at $0°$, $45°$, $90°$, $135°$ and consisting of four Gaussian scales (sigma values of 1, 2, 4 and 8 pixels), resulting in a bank of 16 filters. Mackiewicz also addresses the problem of air bubbles as these can cause problems when attempting to identify frames containing blood because the healthy tissue colour distribution seen through the air bubble is similar to the blood colour distribution, thus triggering false positives. He observed that air bubbles often contain specularities which can be detected using an approach due to Ortiz and Torres [37].

Vilarino et al. [33–35] as well as Igual et al. [38] studied detection of intestinal contractions and intestinal motility disfunction. Villarino claim a sensitivity of 70 % in respect of their approach which involves the analysis of textural, colour and blob features using a Support Vector Machine (SVM).

Recently, Li and Meng [20] proposed a method of bleeding and ulceration detection by means of chromaticity moments constructed from the Tchebichef polynomials. The authors divide the circular CE image into a grid of 36 non-overlapping blocks (30×30 pixels) (similar grid was also used for feature extraction in [12], see Fig. 4), from which they calculate six chromaticity moments. Next, they performed an experiment in which 5400 (1800 normal, 1800 bleeding and 1800 ulceration) image blocks were selected from 300 non-consecutive CE images extracted from 10 patient video sequences. The blocks were randomised and classified using an MLP Neural Network. Finally, the authors reported sensitivity and specificity figures obtained from the block classifications. This was a preliminary study that was not performed on the full length videos.

More recently, Li et al. [22] presented a study with an aim to develop a computer aided system to diagnose small bowel tumours. They proposed a textural feature that is built on wavelet and local binary pattern. They employed a classifier ensemble consisting of k-nearest-neighbor, multilayer perceptron neural network and support vector machine. Results obtained from the single image classification of 600 normal and 600 abnormal capsule images showed the promising performance for small bowel tumour detection.

4 Viewing Speed

Attempts to automatically adapt the viewer's focus of attention based on video content have focused on automatically adjusting the viewing speed and filtering of non-informative frames. Hai et al. [39] proposed video speed is adjusted by an algorithm which plays the video at high speed in stable regions and at slower speed where significant changes between frames occur, signifying the possibility of pathologies. The authors divide each frame into 64 blocks and measure the similarity of colours between respective blocks in consecutive frames. RGB histograms quantized to 163 bins are used to describe each image block. The distance between local histograms is computed using the L1 norm, formally:

$$D_{blk}(i) = \sum_{k=1}^{nbins} \left(\left\| H_{R,k}^n - H_{R,k}^{n+1} \right\| + \left\| H_{G,k}^n - H_{G,k}^{n+1} \right\| + \left\| H_{B,k}^n - H_{B,k}^{n+1} \right\| \right)$$

which is later used to calculate the similarity between two frames:

$$Sim(n) = \frac{1}{n_{blocks}} \sum_{i=1}^{N_{blocks}} sim\_block(i)$$

where

$$sim\_block(i) = \begin{cases} 1: & D_{blk}(i) > Thresh_{block} \\ 0: & otherwise \end{cases}$$

These features are used together with estimates of motion displacement to classify the frame in one of four states and these in turn adjust a delay which controls the speed at which frames are presented to the viewer. The authors conclude that using their method the viewing time may be reduced from 2h to around 30 minutes without 'loss of information'.

The software supplied by both Given Imaging (Rapid Reader) and Olympus (EndoView) also include play speed control. Unfortunately, the details of these algorithms remain unknown. Moreover, in the more recent versions of Given's Rapid Reader, the clinician is given an option of watching a video in either "Normal Mode" or in the "Quick View Mode". Although the "Quick View" mechanism is not precisely explained in the documentation, we noticed that it uses an approach similar to that described above to reduce the viewing time of the video. It must be added though, that the "Quick View" mode skips some frames, displaying only the most suspicious (at least to the algorithm that is used by Given Imaging), which makes it different to the algorithms described above.

The obvious conclusion regarding these methods must be that they are highly subjective. All research on this topic has to include particularly extensive clinical evaluations in order to make sure that the increase in the viewing speed does not increase the number of false negatives [40].

5 Future Directions for CE Research

In a recent review of ten years of CE, Mackiewicz [41] considers a number of exciting opportunities for further research in the field CE video analysis. Firstly, there is the possibility of focusing on specific pathological events possibly addressed by some of the specialist capsules now being marketed (e.g. *PillCam ESO* and *Pill-Cam COLON*). Adaptive control of the speed at which the video is reviewed is also a promising area as it draws from experience gained in other research in the field of video summarization and beyond this, there is the possibility of tools for automated reporting and annotation of CE video. The prospect of more advanced capsules which might be controlled by the physician are probably no more than a decade away. One of the main challenges for CE research is in providing sufficient quantities of annotated training data to enable classifiers to be built. Given that a typical CE exam may contain around 50,000 images, but only a few abnormal events, a reasonably conservative figure for a training set might be 100 exams (about 50 hours of video). The fact that few researchers have access to a database of this size probably explains the lack of significant progress in the field, even following the publication of hundreds of individual papers.

6 Discussion

All of the significant investigators of CE video analysis [12, 21, 27] have used colour and texture features. The preferred colour feature is the HSI colour histogram, encoded using the Haar (MPEG-7) or hybrid (DCT + PCA) transform. Many researchers chose MPEG-7 features, possibly due to the freely available reference software [42], the established track record of these techniques in other content based image retrieval applications, and the work due to Coimbra et al. [25]. All researchers agree that colour texture is a very important component. The groups using MPEG-7 favour the HT descriptor, based on the Gabor wavelet. However, the comparative success of other methods such as LBP adopted by Mackiewicz in an implementation developed by colleagues Connah and Finlayson [14], suggests that the MPEG-7 descriptors may not be the most suitable for this purpose. A number of classifiers have been tested using both feature sets and there is widespread agreement that the Support Vector Classifier yields marginally better results than other methods.

Evaluation of the approaches varies considerably and the lack of a large reference data set is a major drawback. The quality of evaluations undertaken by groups in Norwich, Porto, HongKong and Barcelona is largely due to the support by collaborators at local hospitals or manufacturers. Manufacturers Given Imaging, Olympus and OMOM (jinshangroup.com) all provide example CE video data but primarily motivated by a desire to promote sales, marketing, and training rather than support the development of algorithms by the wider scientific community. The availability of CE video has made a significant impact on the medical imaging community since its introduction in 2001 and there is no doubt that it will become increasingly important, as the number of CE examinations grows.

References

1. Iddan G, Meron G, Glukhovsky A, Swain P (2000) Wireless capsule endoscopy. Nature 405:725–729
2. Ravens AF, Swain P (2002) The wireless capsule: new light in the darkness. Dig Dis 20:127–133
3. Swain M, Ballard D (1991) Color indexing. Int J of Computer Vision 11–32
4. Cox J (2005) Finding blood in capsule endoscopy. Master's thesis, The University of Texas at Arlington
5. Bourbakis N, Makrogiannis S, Kavraki D (2005) A neural network-based detection of bleeding in sequences of WCE images. In: Proceedings of the 5th IEEE symposium on bioinformatics and bioengineering (BIBE'05)
6. Hwang S, Oh J, Tang SJ (2006) Expectation maximization based bleeding detection for wireless capsule endoscopy (WCE) images. In: Proceedings of SPIE, vol 6144, pp 577–587
7. Berens J (2002) Image indexing using compressed colour histograms. PhD thesis, School of Information Systems, University of East Anglia, Norwich, UK
8. Berens J, Finlayson GD, Qiu G (2000) Image indexing using compressed colour histograms. IEE Proc, Vis Image Signal Process 147(4):349–354
9. Berens J, Finlayson GD (2002) An efficient coding of three dimensional colour distributions for image retrieval. In: CIVR2002. Lecture notes in computer science, vol 2383, pp 245–252
10. Berens J, Mackiewicz M, Bell GD (2005) Stomach, intestine and colon tissue discriminators for wireless capsule endoscopy (WCE) images. In: Proceedings of SPIE, vol 5747, pp 283–290
11. Berens J, Mackiewicz M, Fisher M, Bell GD (2005) Using colour distributions to discriminate tissues in wireless capsule endoscopy images. In: Proceedings of medical image understanding and analyses 2005 conference, Bristol, UK, July 2005, pp 107–110
12. Mackiewicz M, Berens J, Fisher M (2008) Wireless capsule endoscopy colour video segmentation. IEEE Trans Med Imaging 27(12):1769–1781
13. Mackiewicz M (2007) Computer-assisted wireless capsule endoscopy video analysis. PhD thesis, School of Computing Sciences, University of East Anglia, Norwich, UK
14. Connah D, Finlayson GD (2006) Using local binary pattern operators for colour constant image indexing. In: CGIV 2006 conference proceedings
15. Ojala T, Pietikäinen M, Mäenpää T (2002) Multiresolution gray-scale and rotation invariant texture classification with local binary patterns. IEEE Trans Pattern Anal Mach Intell 24(7):971–987
16. Mäenpää T, Pietikäinen M (2004) Classification with color and texture: jointly or separately. Pattern Recognit 37:1629–1640
17. Pietikäinen M, Hadid A, Zhao G, Ahonen T (2011) Computer vision using local binary patterns. Springer, Berlin

18. Berens J, Finlayson GD (2002) An efficient coding of three dimensional colour distributions for image retrieval. In: Proc. CIVR2002. Lecture notes in computer science, vol 2383, pp 245–252

19. Lee J, Oh J, Shah SK, Yuan X, Tang SJ (2007) Automatic classification of digestive organs in wireless capsule endoscopy videos. In: Proceedings of the 2007 ACM symposium on applied computing, SAC'07. ACM, New York, pp 1041–1045

20. Li B, Meng MQ-H (2009) Computer-based detection of bleeding and ulcer in wireless capsule endoscopy images by chromaticity moments. Comput Biol Med 39:141–147

21. Li B, Meng MQ-H (2009) Computer-aided detection of bleeding regions for capsule endoscopy images. IEEE Trans Biomed Eng 56(4):1032–1039

22. Li B, Meng MQ-H, Lau JYW (2011) Computer-aided small bowel tumor detection for capsule endoscopy. Artif Intell Med 52(1):11–16

23. Coimbra M, Campos P, Silva Cunha JP (2005) Extracting clinical information from endoscopic capsules exams using MPEG-7 visual descriptors. In: 2nd European workshop on the integration of knowledge semantic and digital media technologies, November 2005. IEE, New York

24. Coimbra M, Campos P, Silva Cunha JP (2006) Topographic segmentation and transit times estimation for endoscopic capsule exams. In: Proceedings of the IEEE international conference on acoustics, speech, and signal processing, vol II, Toulouse, France, May 2006, pp 1164–1167

25. Coimbra M, Campos P, Silva Cunha JP (2006) MPEG-7 visual descriptors—contributions for automated feature extraction in capsule endoscopy. IEEE Trans Circuits Syst Video Technol 16:628–637

26. Coimbra M, Kustra J, Silva Cunha JP, Campos P (2006) Combining color with spatial and temporal position of the endoscopic capsule for improved topographic classification and segmentation. In: Proceedings of the 1st international conference on semantic and digital media technologies, Athens, Greece, December 2006

27. Silva Cunha JP, Coimbra M, Campos P, Soares JM (2008) Automated topographic segmentation and transit time estimation in endoscopic capsule exams. IEEE Trans Medical Imaging 27(1):19–27

28. Chang S-F, Sikora T, Puri A (2001) Overview of the MPEG-7 standard. IEEE Trans Circuits Syst Video Technol 11(6):688–695. Special issue on MPEG-7

29. Manjunath BS, Ohm J-R, Vasudevan VV, Yamada A (2001) Color and texture descriptors. IEEE Trans Circuits Syst Video Technol 11(6):703–715

30. Wu P, Ro YM, Won CS, Choi Y (2001) Texture descriptors in MPEG-7. In: Skarbek W (ed) Proceedings CAIP 2001. LNCS, vol 2124, pp 21–28

31. Duda K, Zielinski T, Fraczek R, Bulat J, Duplaga M (2007) Localization of endoscopic capsule in the GI tract based on MPEG-7 visual descriptors. In: IEEE international workshop on imaging systems and techniques, IST'07, May 2007, pp 1–4

32. Duda K, Zielinski T, Duplaga M, Grega M, Leszczuk M (2007) VQ classification based on MPEG-7 visual descriptors for video endoscopic capsule localisation in the gastrointestinal tract. In: 15th European signal processing conference (EUSIPCO 2007), Poznan, Poland, September 2007

33. Vilarino F, Kuncheva LI, Radeva P (2005) ROC curves and video analysis optimization in intestinal capsule endoscopy. Pattern Recognit Lett, Special Issue on ROC analysis

34. Vilarino F, Spyridonos P, Puyol O, Vitrià J, Radeva P (2006) Automatic detection of intestinal juices in wireless capsule video endoscopy. In: Proceedings of ICPR, pp 531–537

35. Vilarino F, Spyridonos P, DeIorio F, Vitrià J, Azpiroz F, Radeva P (2010) Intestinal motility assessment with video capsule endoscopy: automatic annotation of phasic intestinal contractions. IEEE Trans Med Imaging 29(2):246–259

36. Mackiewicz M, Fisher M, Jamieson C (2008) Bleeding detection in wireless capsule endoscopy using adaptive colour histogram model and support vector classification. In: Proceedings of SPIE, vol 6914

37. Ortiz F, Torres F (2006) Automatic detection and elimination of specular reflectance in color images by means of MS diagram and vector connected filters. IEEE Trans Syst, Man, Cybern, Part C 36(5):681–687
38. Igual L, Seguí S, Vitrià J, Azpiroz F, Radeva P (2007) Eigenmotion-based detection of intestinal contractions. Lect Notes Comput Sci 4673(2007):293–300
39. Hai V, Echigo T, Sagawa R, Yagi K, Schiba M, Higuchi K, Arakawa T, Yagi Y (2006) Adaptive control of video display for diagnostic assistance by analysis of capsule endoscopic images. In: Proceedings of ICPR, pp 531–537
40. Zheng Y, Hawkins L, Wolff J, Goloubeva O, Goldberg E (2012) Detection of lesions during capsule endoscopy: physician performance is disappointing. Am J Gastroenterol
41. Mackiewicz M (2011) Capsule endoscopy—state of the technology and computer vision tools after the first decade. In: Pascu O (ed) New techniques in gastrointestinal endoscopy. InTech, New York
42. Multimedia content description interfaces. Part 6: reference software. MPEG-7 ISO/IEC 15938-6, 2003

Automated Prototype Generation for Multi-color Karyotyping

Xuqing Wu, Shishir Shah, and Fatima Merchant

Abstract This chapter presents an algorithm for automatically generating a proto-type from multicolor karyotypes obtained via multi-spectral imaging of human chro-mosomes. The single representative prototype of the color karyotype that is gener-ated represents the analytical integration of a group of karyotypes obtained via Mul-ticolor Fluorescence In Situ Hybridization (MFISH) method. Multicolor karyotyp-ing is a 24-color MFISH method that allows simultaneous screening of the genome. It allows for the detection of a wide variety of anomalies in human chromosomes, including subtle and complex rearrangements. Although, multicolor karyotyping al-lows visual detection of gross anomalies, misclassified pixels make manual exam-ination difficult. Additionally, in the absence of prior knowledge of the anomaly, interpretation of the karyotypes can be ambiguous. In this study we have developed an automated method for the generation of a single representative prototype of the color karyotype, which assists the screening of chromosomal aberrations by compu-tational removal of non-physiological anomalies. We hypothesize that generation of a single representative prototype of the color karyotype from multiple karyotypes (k) for a given specimen can highlight all the aberrations, while minimizing misclassi-fied pixels arising from inconsistencies in sample preparation, hybridization and imaging procedures. A three-tier approach is implemented to achieve the generation of the representative color karyotype from a set of multiple (>2) karyotypes. The first step involves the automated extraction of individual chromosomes from each karyotype in the set, followed by chromosome straightening and size normaliza-tion. In the second step, the extracted and normalized chromosomes belonging to each of the 24 color classes are automatically assigned to a particular group (1, 2, 3, etc.) based on the ploidy level (monoploid, diploid, triploid, etc.), respectively. For automated group assignment, Bayesian classification is utilized to determine the probability that a particular chromosome belongs to a specific group based on the similarity between the chromosomes within the group. Similarity is evaluated

X. Wu · S. Shah · F. Merchant (✉)
Department of Computer Science, University of Houston, Houston, TX 77204, USA
e-mail: fmerchan@Central.UH.EDU

F. Merchant
Department of Engineering Technology, University of Houston, Houston, TX 77204, USA

M.E. Celebi, G. Schaefer (eds.), *Color Medical Image Analysis*,
Lecture Notes in Computational Vision and Biomechanics 6,
DOI 10.1007/978-94-007-5389-1_8, © Springer Science+Business Media Dordrecht 2013

using two distance metrics: (1) two-dimensional (2D) histogram based descriptors, and (2) Eigen space representation based on Principal Component Analysis (PCA). Finally in the third step, we compute the prototype of the color karyotype by generating the representative chromosome for each group in the 24 color classes using pixel-based fusion. This approach allows us to generate the representative prototype color karyotype that reflects all anomalies for a given specimen, while rejecting non-physiological inconsistencies. Furthermore, automation not only reduces the workload, but also allows alleviation of subjectivity by providing a quantitative formulation based on statistical analysis.

1 Introduction

A karyotype is a pictorial presentation of all the chromosomes in a genome, wherein homologous metaphase chromosomes are displayed as groups in standard classes (categories). In humans, a normal karyotype includes 46 chromosomes that are categorized into a total of 23 classes, of which classes 1 to 22 consists of pairs of homologous chromosomes, and the final class includes the sex chromosome pair of either XX for a female or XY for a male [1]. Clinicians routinely use karyotypes to diagnose cancers and genetic diseases [2–8]. Two approaches are widely used for generating karyotypes, namely, G-banding [7] and color karyotyping [2, 9].

G-banding involves the use of the Giemsa dye that binds DNA and produces characteristic and reproducible banding patterns for individual chromosomes. These banding patterns are then used to identify and group homologous pairs of chromosomes in a karyotype, which enables cytogeneticists to recognize the differences between chromosomes and to link different disease phenotypes to chromosomal anomalies. G-banded karyotypes are gray-scale visualizations of the number and appearance of chromosomes in a species. Manual interpretation requires knowledge of the unique banding patterns for each of the 24 chromosomes and thus entails considerable operator training and experience.

In contrast, color karyotypes represent the chromosomes in 24 unique colors. Color karyotyping is a molecular cytogenetic technique that is popularly used for studying complex inter-chromosomal rearrangements in cancer. Chromosomes are first labeled with finite numbers of spectrally distinct fluorophores in a combinatorial fashion, such that each homologous pair of chromosomes is uniquely labeled [10, 11]. Next, dedicated spectral imaging microscopes are used to capture images of each fluorophore, and the acquired images are computationally analyzed to enable the classification of individual chromosomes based on the combinatorial labeling scheme of probes. Based on the mechanisms of spectral image acquisition and classification, color karyotyping is broadly categorized into spectral karyotyping (SKY; uses interferometer-based spectral imaging) [12] or multiplex FISH (M-FISH; uses fluorochrome-specific optical filters) [13]. The generated color karyotype allows the visualization of individual chromosomes in a unique color, thereby permitting rapid visual and qualitative resolution of structural and numerical chromosome abnormalities. This is an advantage over G-banded karyotypes in which certain chromosomal aberrations, in the absence of specialized training cannot be easily and unequivocally identified by visualization of the alternating dark and light chromosome bands [14]. Disadvantages of color karyotyping include the inability to (1) define the translocation breakpoints, and (2) detect intrachromosomal rearrangements because they do not result in a color change along the chromosome.

Although several studies have demonstrated that both SKY and M-FISH systems are highly accurate in identifying chromosomal aberrations [15–18], inherent limitations of these methods demand careful interpretation of the karyotypic information. Pixel classification can be poor due to low signal to noise ratio in the images resulting from autofluorescence and non-uniform hybridization. Additionally it has been shown that "Fluorescence flaring" [19] frequently results in misclassified pixels that can lead to erroneous interpretations at chromosome overlaps, translocation breakpoints, and chromosomal regions containing co-amplified material [19–21]. As compared to interpreting G-banded karyotypes, anomaly detection is relatively easier in color karyotypes because of the ease in identifying areas where a chromosome, painted in one color, has a small piece of a different chromosome, painted in another color, attached to it. However, in order to screen chromosomal rearrangements, cytogeneticists not only have to confirm the chromosome classification, but also need to flag all the possible anomalies. This information cannot be ascertained based on a single metaphase, and a multi-cell approach is necessary. Interpretation of anomalies is further confounded when the decision has to be based on the examination of multiple karyotypes that typically display inter-karyotype variability and often intra-karyotype variability of the classified chromosomes due to the presence of misclassified color pixels. Thus, we have developed an automated approach that allows alleviation of certain ambiguities such as misclassified and overlapping pixels that are inherent to color karyotyping.

Our approach leverages the fact that using multi-cell metaphase karyotypes for genetic screening can highlight the differences generated between two homologous chromosomes due to technical artifacts and that such differences can be resolved by analyzing multiple karyotypes from one individual. It is highly unlikely that the same technical artifact would occur repeatedly in a given specimen and thus can be computationally resolved by the examination of the color information at each pixel from multiple chromosomes of the same class. Although performing such an examination manually is not practical, it is not only computationally feasible but can also be statistically corroborated.

Although the prototype representation of the color karyotype introduced in this study will directly benefit the visual screening of chromosome aberrations, it has the ability to allow an informed screening process since prototype creation is founded on statistical analysis of the frequency of occurrence of each colored pixel in each chromosome computed over multiple karyotypes. Currently, other than the conventional manual viewing of multiple karyotypes for each subject, there is no computational approach that facilitates screening of anomalies from M-FISH/SKY karyotypes. To the best of our knowledge, the only other approach that assists visualization of color karyotypes is the computer generated SKYGRAM image, which consists of a colored ideogram where each chromosome in the karyotype is displayed in its unique SKY classification color, with band overlay. The SKYGRAM image is only available for images in SKY/CGH database [22], and requires information on the start (top) and stop (bottom) band for each various segments on the chromosome, which is not typically available for studies that comprise solely of color karyotyping. We describe here for the first time, an approach for visualizing chromosomal aberrations in color karyotype via generation of a unique pictorial representative prototype that embeds information from multiple karyotypes.

2 Overview of Methodology

Each karyotype in a normal individual has 22 pairs of autosomal chromosomes and one pair of sex chromosomes, resulting in a total of 24 classes of chromosome. The number of copies of chromosomes in each class is dependent on the ploidy level, which can either by normal (two copies) or abnormal (one, three, four, etc.). The problem of generating a representative karyotype given multiple karyotypes can be viewed as one of image fusion, where multiple images for each chromosome are examined to generate a single view that mirrors the aggregate information based on the dominant consensus from the multiple chromosomes.

To fulfill this objective in an automated manner, the primary aim is to enable an approach to cluster or group chromosomes such that for each class, homologous chromosomes are assigned to a specific group (1, 2, 3, etc.), where chromosomes within a given group exhibit maximal similarity. Here similarity is related to comparing the spatial distribution of colors along each chromosome. Determining positional occurrence of color is critical in order to differentiate true chromosomal aberrations from color inconsistencies arising due to sample processing and image acquisition. Since each karyotype is classified independently, the arrangement of all copies of a chromosome in a given class may not be consistent across all karyotypes. For example, consider six karyotypes where one copy of the pair of homologous chromosomes in class 1 has a translocation. This would appear as a chromosome pair where one of the chromosomes has a uniform unique color while the other copy shows two colors. For a prototype karyotype, the chromosome copies in each of the six karyotypes should be fused into a single pair where one has a uniform color whereas the other has two colors. In order to achieve this, the 12 chromosomes of class 1 from the 6 karyotypes have to be appropriately grouped such that all the chromosome copies with the translocation are in the same group, whereas the normal copies are in the second group. Hence, before we can perform fusion of individual chromosome images, we have to organize the chromosome copies from the multiple karyotypes to be consistently segregated into appropriate groups (determined by the ploidy level).

Figure 1 presents a flowchart of our processing pipeline. Initially all chromosomes are extracted from individual color karyotypes, straightened and normalized to a standard size. Next based on a priori information on the total number of karyotypes, the chromosomes are grouped such that the homologous pairs of chromosomes from the multiple karyotypes are assigned to different groups based on their

Fig. 1 Flowchart illustrating the processing pipeline for automatic generation of prototypes

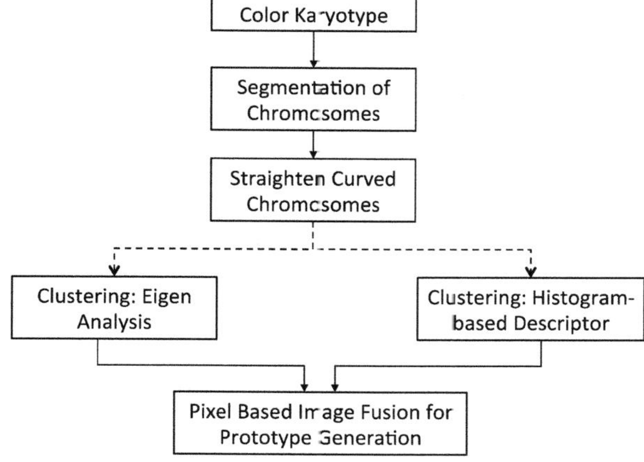

constitutive color pixel population. To do so, two methods are evaluated, each assuming a different descriptive model for the spatial distribution of constitutive colored pixels on each chromosome. First a histogram-based approach is used that performs grouping based on maximizing the similarity of spatial distribution of the colored pixels across chromosomes within a group. Second, a PCA-based approach is used that aims to minimize variability of the dominant colors within chromosomes in a group. Both approaches follow a Bayesian classification framework to group homologous chromosomes (for each one of the 24 classes) across multiple karyotypes into multiple groups (depending on ploidy level) based on the similarity of color and position of the constitutive pixels in each chromosome. For example in case of euploidy, chromosomes for each class are assigned to the most similar one of the two groups. Following segregation of all chromosomes, we compute the final prototype chromosome by pixel-based fusion. Since each pixel can take one of 24 colors, we generate an ordered set of pixels for every position (x, y) across all k chromosomes. We then compute the mode of the ordered set. For fusion, we use a simple selection criterion based on a threshold that provides a lower bound on the frequency of observing a specific color. If a color value varies from the mode, the pixel is assigned a value of zero (color is uncertain). The methodology is described in detail in the following sections.

3 Methods

A three-tier approach is implemented to achieve the generation of the representative color karyotype from a set of multiple (>2) karyotypes. The steps include chromosome extraction and normalization, chromosome grouping and pixel-based fusion for prototype generation.

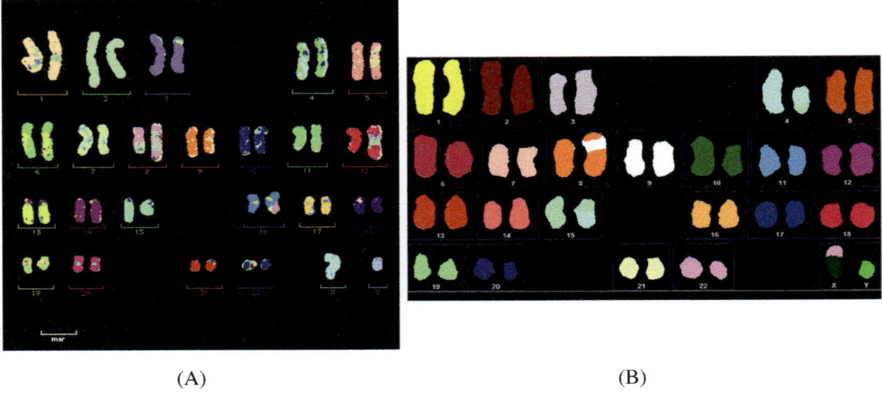

(A)   (B)

Fig. 2 (**A**) Representative color karyotype from a M-FISH system. (**B**) Representative color karyotype from a SKY system

3.1 Chromosome Extraction, Straightening and Size Normalization

The first step in the algorithm is to automatically extract chromosomes from a fully annotated and finalized karyotype. Color karyotypes for both M-FISH and SKY are typically presented in a standardized format. For example, Fig. 2(A, B) presents a sample color karyotype from a M-FISH [15] and SKY system [2].

As seen in the color karyotypes, homologous chromosome pairs for each class are arranged in an ordered sequence from 1–24. Moreover, each class is further separated from the neighboring classes. This systematic ordered spatial arrangement allows for individual chromosomes to be easily extracted from the karyotypes via sequential cropping of the chromosome sub-images based on position and class color.

Following extraction of the chromosome sub-image, the next step comprises of chromosome straightening [23, 24]. Chromosomes are naturally flexible, and metaphase chromosomes are typically visualized not only in a variety of sizes and lengths, but can also appear to be bent or curved in shape. We implemented the following algorithm to straighten curved chromosomes. Initially, the morphological medial axis transformation is applied to the binary image of the chromosome to identify the central axis of the curved chromosome [25]. Next, the central axis is smoothed using a two-dimensional cubic spline function. For any given point on the smoothed central axis, we determine the normal direction of the tangent line and find the intersection of the normal line and the two outermost edges of the original curved chromosome. For any point along the central axis, pixels identified on the normal line are mapped onto a new chromosome image such that the central axis is vertically straightened at an angle of 90°, and the normal line at each pixel on the central axis is now horizontally oriented (i.e. at an angle of 0°) perpendicular to the vertical. The final straightened chromosome image is obtained by repeating this

Fig. 3 Results of
chromosome straightening

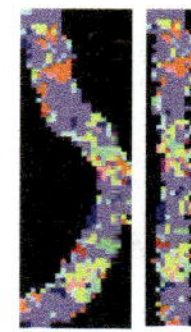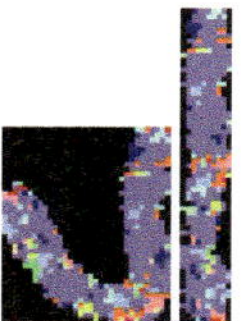

step for each point (i.e. straightening the normal line) along the central axis. Figure 3 shows representative images of curved chromosomes and the resulting straightened chromosomes.

Finally, the last pre-processing step was normalization of chromosome size in terms of length and width. This step is necessitated to standardize the chromosomes in order to enable further processing steps related to grouping and pixel-based fusion for prototype generation. Size normalization across the length and width was achieved via pixel resampling (up/down-sampling) [26]. As a rule, size determination was based on selecting the dimensions to match that of the largest chromosome in the set of karyotypes being analyzed.

3.2 Clustering Approach for Assigning Homologous Chromosomes to Ploidy-Level Based Groups

Each karyotype in a normal individual has 22 pairs of autosomal chromosomes and one pair of sex chromosomes. To be able to extract the prototype from multiple karyotypes, copies of chromosomes for each of the 24 classes from all the karyotypes need to be correctly segregated and grouped based on the spatial distribution of their constitutive colors. We pose this as a chromosome-grouping problem. For example, given a chromosome from a specific class, we identify its multiple copies with the labels $L_1, \ldots, L_p$, where $p =$ ploidy level for the chromosome class. Let $K = 1, \ldots, N$ denote the number of karyotypes. Thus, for any chromosome class in the genome, the total copies in a karyotype can be denoted by $C_{l,k} = \{c_{1,k}, c_{2,k}, \ldots, c_{p,k}\}$. Further, the total number of possible chromosome grouping combinations for a given class would be p^K. For a given number of karyotypes and the ploidy level for each chromosome class, the number of groups is thus fixed and can be denoted as $G = \{G_1, G_2, \ldots, G_{p^k}\}$. In this case, the identification of the group that constitutes the correct labels for each of the chromosome can be considered a classification problem.

Consider R to be a chromosome randomly chosen from a group in G. Excluding the group corresponding to the sampled chromosome, the remaining groups can be denoted as $\hat{G} = \{G_1, \ldots, G_{(p^{k-1})}\}$. The probability of the random sample R belonging to a group G_k from $\hat{G}$ can be calculated as per the Bayesian decision rule as

$$P(G_k|R) = \frac{P(R|G_k) * P(G_k)}{P(R)}$$

where $P(R) = \sum_{k=1}^{M} P(R|G_k) * P(G_k)$ and $M = p^{K-1}$.

Thus, the true assignment of labels can be calculated based on maximizing the posterior probability,

$$P(\hat{G}|R) = \arg\max_{k} P(G_k|R).$$

However, since we have no a priori knowledge of the true groups from which a sample is chosen and the denominator is typically constant for a given known set of groups, the assignment of the randomly chosen chromosome into one of the groups can be simplified to the estimation of the maximum likelihood such that:

$$P(R|\hat{G}) = \arg\max_{k} P(R|G_k).$$

This suggests that each group can be best represented by observations R with the correct label assignments. Thus, if Q independent observations are sampled resulting in an observation set O, the joint conditional distribution function over all observations can be written as:

$$P(O|\hat{G}) = \prod_{k=1}^{Q} P(R_k|\hat{G}).$$

The formulation can be further simplified by maximizing the log-likelihood such that,

$$\Gamma\{R_1, R_2, \ldots, R_Q|\hat{G}\} = \sum_{k=1}^{Q} \log P(R_k|\hat{G})$$

where $P(R_k|\hat{G})$ defines the probability of assigning R_k to the group $\hat{G}$, and can be measured by the distance between the sample R_k and the group center $C_{\hat{G}}$. In this study, $P(R_k|\hat{G})$ is estimated as:

$$P(R_k|\hat{G}) \propto \frac{1}{\|R_k - C_{\hat{G}}\|}.$$

3.2.1 Distance Metrics for Bayesian Classification

Two approaches were evaluated to compute the distance metric $\|R_k - C_{\hat{G}}\|$ for Bayesian classification. In doing so, the two key elements needed are the ability to find an appropriate representation for chromosomes R_k and a corresponding mechanism to define the group center $C_{\hat{G}}$.

3.2.2 Two-Dimensional (2D) Histogram Based Descriptors

To facilitate the computation of the distance metric, cropped images of chromosomes were represented by histogram based local descriptors. Specifically, 2D image signatures were generated to accurately represent the color content of the chromosome with respect to its spatial distribution within the chromosome. The 2D

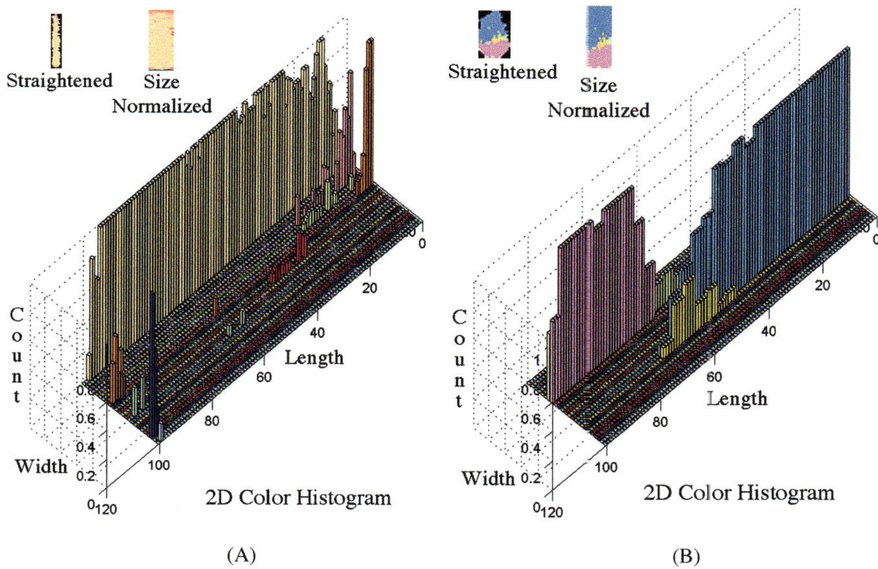

Fig. 4 Size normalized chromosome image and its 2D Color Histogram. (**A**) Chromosome with few misclassified pixels. (**B**) Chromosome with a terminal translocation

histogram was used to represent the signature of each size normalized chromosome image. For each image with the size of $m \times n$, we generated the $m \times 24$ 2D histogram. So each line of the image is represented by a 24-bin 1D histogram.

Figure 4 presents examples of 2D color histograms for (A) a chromosome with few misclassified pixels, and (B) a chromosome with a terminal translocation. As seen in Fig. 4, the 2D histogram provides a clear visualization of the spatial distribution of the different colors within the chromosome. In the case of the chromosome with few misclassified pixels (Fig. 4A), the unique color of the chromosome (peach) predominates the entire length of the chromosome, whereas for the chromosome with the terminal translocation (Fig. 4A), the two different colors; blue and pink; dominate at the two opposite ends along the length of the chromosome. Thus, the 2D color histogram may be used to differentiate chromosomes based on the spatial localization of its constitutive colors.

The distance between any two 2D histograms (i.e. $\| R_k - C_{\hat{G}} \|$) is then determined as follows. First, we calculate the Hellinger distance between each pair of corresponding 1D histograms [27], whose result is saved in an $m \times 1$ vector. Then, the final distance between the 2D histograms is measured by the L2 norm of the vector. To search for the maximum likelihood for optimal label assignments ($\arg\max_k P(R|G_k)$), we use a variant of k-means classification to define group centers. For K karyotypes and each chromosome class with p being the ploidy level, each sampled chromosome needs to be evaluated for assignment into one of the p^{K-1} groups. For each group, the group center is defined by computing an average 2D histogram from all the chromosomes in that group. The assignment of the sampled chromosome into one of the groups is based on computing the distance defined above. A total group score is computed by taking the product of distances between the sampled chromosome and all group centers. Once the initial grouping is done, we recalculate the new averages based on all 2D histograms in the group and note it to be the new group center. For each of the groups, we select the chromosome that is furthest from the group center and use it as the new sample. The above steps are repeated until a minimum total group score is obtained.

3.2.3 Eigen Space Representation

An alternate approach to measuring similarity or distance between chromosomes within a group is to measure similarity within a linear subspace of the images. One such subspace can be defined by the eigenvectors of the images within a group. Hence, the distance between two images can be measured in eigenspace, within which a chromosome image can be represented based on the principal components $\{u_j\}$ that best describes the covariance across another group of images.

Consider one of the groups G_k comprising of I_i, $i = 1, \ldots, z$ images. A matrix A is formed where each column of the matrix is one of the vectorized images. Thus, for images of size $m \times n$, the matrix A is of size $mn \times z$. The eigenvectors are determined based on singular value decomposition, as follows:

$$A = USV^T$$

where the columns of U are eigenvectors of AA^T. Any image I_i can be recovered as follows:

$$I_i = \sum_{j=1}^{z-1} u_j s_j v_{(i,j)}$$

$$I_i = \sum_{j=1}^{z-1} w_{(i,j)} u_j$$

where s_j is the jth singular value, $v_{(i,j)}$ is the ith element of the jth eigenvector in V and $w(i, j) = \frac{\langle a_i, u_j \rangle}{s_j}$. The set of coefficients $w(i, j)$, $j = 1, \ldots, z$ can be summarized into a z dimensional vector w_i, and the distance between any two images (i, j) can be estimated as $\|w_i - w_j\|$. Optimal group assignments for each sampled chromosome is then obtained through an exhaustive minimization of the distance across all groups.

3.3 Prototype Generation Using Pixel-Based Fusion

Comparison of each pixel amongst all the chromosomes in the same group was used to create the final prototype image for each chromosome. The color for each pixel was chosen based on the majority vote from all karyotypes. Thus, pixels that had the same color across chromosomes from all the karyotypes in a set retained their original color, whereas other pixels in a chromosome with differing colors across the multiple karyotypes for which a majority vote was not feasible were labeled as misclassified pixels.

Having determined the group of chromosomes with the most similar spatial distribution of colors, we computed the representative chromosome by performing pixel-based fusion. Since each pixel on any chromosome can take one of twenty-four colors, we first generate an ordered set of pixels for every position (x, y) across all k chromosomes. We also compute the mode of the ordered set to determine the value with the largest number of occurrences. We use a simple selection criterion based on a percentage threshold that provides a lower bound on the frequency of observing the color value for the fused chromosome. Given the ordered set A of B pixels at location (x, y), the value to be assigned to the fused representation is given by:

$$F(x, y) = A\{\%Threshold \times B\}.$$

Further, if the color value is not the same as the mode of the ordered set, the pixel value is assigned a value of zero since the true color is uncertain. We set the threshold value to 0.6 to reflect that the mode should comprise of a minimum of 60 % majority across all colors. Figure 5 illustrates the approach for prototype generation.

3.4 Assessment Metrics for Data Analysis

The performance of the algorithm for automatically generating a representative prototype from a set of multiple color karyotypes was assessed using two approaches. First, the representative karyotype was compared to the ground truth, which is the manually annotated karyotype. Second, we determined the color variance between the two clustering approaches to assess their performance. Since, in color karyotyping, each chromosome has a predefined unique color c, any other colors appearing in the chromosome may be regarded as noise. Then the signal to noise ratio SNR for each chromosome can be computed as follows:

$$SNR = \frac{N_{color=c}}{N_{color \neq c}}$$

where $N_{color \neq c}$ is the number of pixels that have color other than the predefined unique color for the given chromosome, and $N_{color=c}$ is the number of pixels with the predefined unique color for the given chromosome. For copies of chromosomes belonging to the same group, SNR should be comparable, and any inconsistencies may be reflected by the variance of SNR, which we denote as the color variance of each group. To compare the grouping performance of the histogram-based method and the eigenspace analysis, we determined the sum of the variance of all the groups

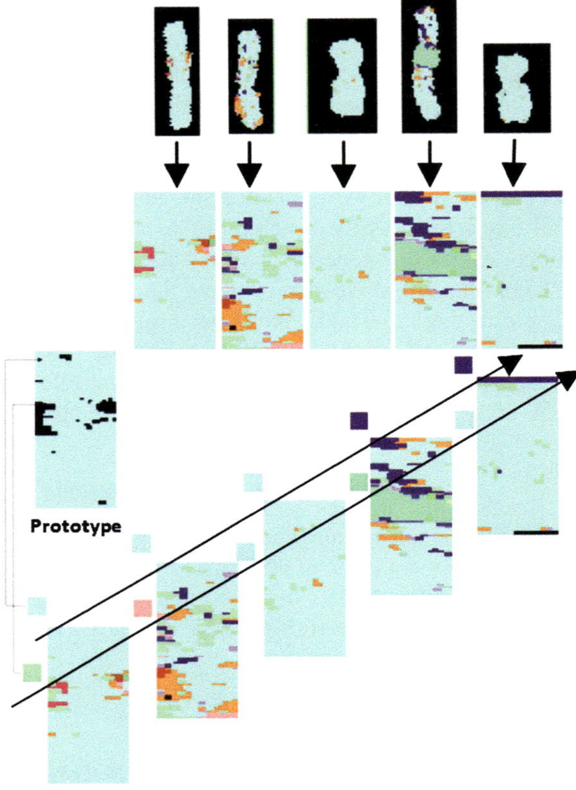

Fig. 5 Prototype generation using majority vote based pixel fusion

for each case analyzed. In addition, we also computed a measure of color purity to understand the inherent quality of karyotypes, defined as:

$$Purity = \frac{N_{color=c}}{N_{pixels}}$$

where N_{pixels} is the total number of pixels on the chromosome. *Purity* is computed for each chromosome and the measure of color purity for a case is taken as the average across all chromosomes.

4 Results

Color karyotype images were randomly selected from the M-FISH Chromosome Imaging Database developed and maintained by the Laboratory for Image and Video Engineering at The University of Texas at Austin [28, 29]. We tested our algorithms using a total of 15 cases, each with multiple color karyotypes. The number of karyotypes in each case ranged from 3–7. Overall, we had 9 cases with

Table 1 List of color karyotype cases analyzed

No	Karyotype	#	Histogram based	GF	Eigen based	GF
1	46, XY	5	46, XY	1	46, XY	1
2	46, XY	6	46, XY	1	46, XY	0.95
3	45, XX, −13	5	45, XX, −13	1	45, XX, −13	0.95
4	46, XY	3	46, XY	1	46, XY	0.95
5	46, XY	7	46, XY	1	46, XX	0.95
6	44, −X, −5, −14, +18, Ins(11; 8), t(15; 16), t(7; 16), t(9; 14), t(14; 15), t(5; 17)	5	44, −X, −5, −14, +18, Ins(11; 8), t(7; 16), t(9; 14), t(14; 15), t(5; 17)	1	44, −X, −5, −14, +18, Ins(11; 8), t(7; 16), t(9; 14), t(14; 15)	0.77
7	46, XX	3	46, XX	1	46, XX	1
8	47, XX, +9	3	47, XX, +9	1	47, XX, +9	1
9	46, XX	4	46, XX	1	46, XX	1
10	46, XY	3	46, XY	1	46, XY	1
11	46, XY	4	46, XY	1	46, XY	1
12	46, XY	3	46, XY	1	46, XY	1
13	46, XX, t(X; 4)	5	46, XX, t(X; 4)	1	46, XX, t(X; 4)	0.95
14	46, XY, t(3; 13), t(8; 3), t(16; 8)	3	46, XY, t(3; 13), t(8; 3), t(16; 8)	1	46, XY, t(3; 13), t(8; 3), t(16; 8)	1
15	45, XY, −18, −22, +11, t(7; 8), t(9; 10), t(11; 20), t(15; 18), t(20; 5)	4	45, XY, −18, −22, +11, t(7; 8), t(9; 10), t(11; 20), t(15; 18), t(20; 5)	0.91	45, XY, −18, −22, +11, t(7; 8), t(9; 10), t(11; 20), t(15; 18), t(20; 5)	0.91

normal karyotypes and the remaining 6 cases included chromosomal aberrations such as aneuploidy, insertions and terminal translocaticns. Table 1 presents a list of the 15 cases analyzed along with information about the specific abnormalities, the number of karyotypes per case, and the results obtained based on manual reading of the generated prototypes. We also report the grouping factor (GF) for the two methods, histogram- and eigen-based grouping. GF is measured based on the correctness of grouping per chromosome. As an example, for a normal karyotype 46, XY, if chromosome X and Y are incorrectly grouped, the resultant GF would be $(46 - 2)/46 = 0.95$. This measure provides an indication of the grouping accuracy between the two methods.

Our results indicate that the histogram-based distance metric is more effective in achieving grouping of similar homologous chromosomes across karyotypes and pixel based fusion can resolve sample processing anomalies such as overlapping chromosomes and misclassified pixels occurring due to cross-hybridization, as well as in detecting chromosomal translocations and insertions that are in the range of 3–50 Mbp and greater. Figure 6 represents the results of grouping chromosomes that have overlaps, random instances of misclassified pixels due to cross-

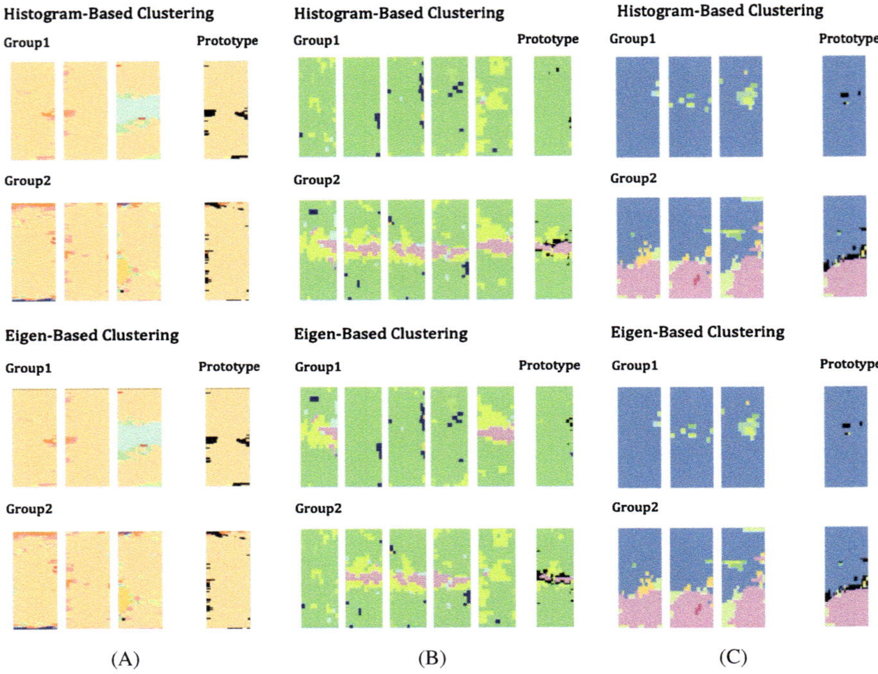

Fig. 6 Results of grouping chromosomes with (**A**) overlaps, (**B**) insertions, (**C**) translocations

hybridization, and physiological translocations. As seen in Fig. 6A, the six chromosomes of class 1 from three karyotypes are effectively clustered into two groups by both the histogram-based and the eigen-based distance metrics, and the pale green region apparent on one of the chromosomes in group1 is effectively removed in the prototype. Similarly, as seen in Fig. 6C the six chromosomes of class 16 from three karyotypes are effectively clustered into two groups wherein the chromosomes with the translocation are all assigned to the appropriate group by both the histogram-based and the eigen-based distance metric. However, although the final prototype image is accurate in Fig. 6B, the eigen-based clustering fails to accurately group all the chromosomes with the internal insertion.

Figure 7 shows a set consisting of six color karyotypes with the classification 46, XY. Figure 8 shows the representative prototypes generated using the two approaches, namely; histogram-based 2D descriptors and eigen-analysis for grouping of chromosomes. As seen in Fig. 8, both the approaches are effective in generating an accurate representative karyotype.

Figure 9 shows a set consisting of four color karyotypes with the classification 45, XY, −18, −22, +11, t(7; 8), t(9; 10), t(11; 20), t(15; 18), t(20; 5). Figure 10 shows the representative prototypes generated using the two approaches, namely; histogram-based 2D descriptors and eigen-analysis for grouping of chromosomes.

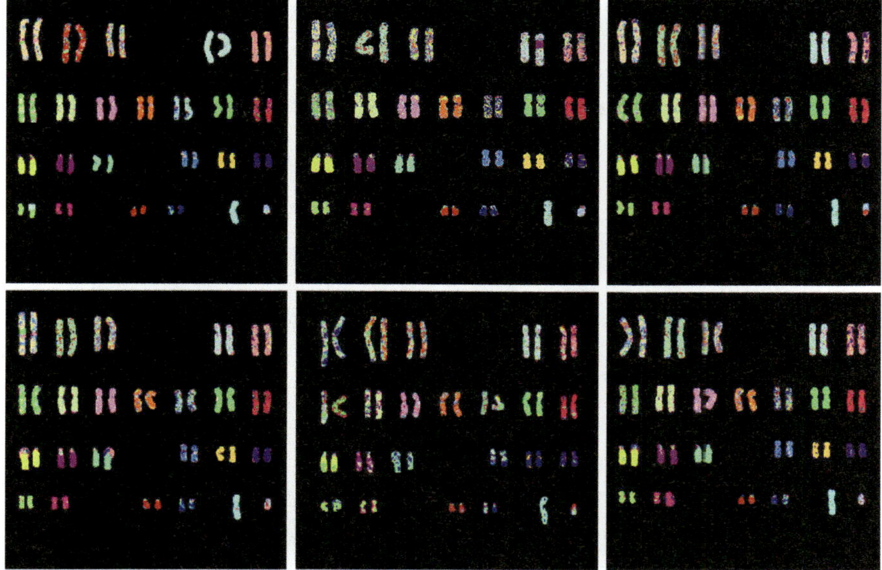

Fig. 7 Six color karyotypes for a single sample case with karyotype 46 XY

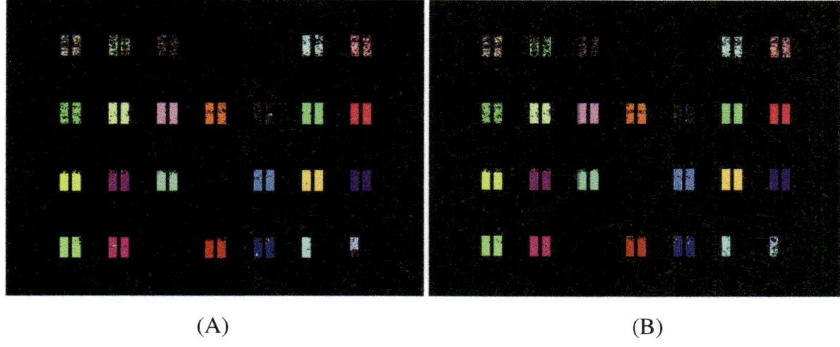

(A)   (B)

Fig. 8 (A) Prototype created by histogram-based. (B) Prototype created by eigen-based method

As seen in Fig. 10, both the approaches are effective in generating an accurate representative karyotype that mirror several chromosomal aberrations.

The prototypes generated by the histogram-based method matched the ground-truth karyotypes in 14 out of the 15 cases analyzed. The only sample where the prototype did not match the ground-truth was case 6 (Table 1) where it missed a t(15; 16), primarily due to the size of the translocation being less than 3 Mbp, which is beyond the detection limit of MFISH. Similarly, the grouping efficiency of the histogram-based approach was 100 % in all but one case (case 15; 91 %). However, this may be attributed to the high color variance (Fig. 11) and moderate purity of the karyotypes in the sample set (Fig. 12; lower values indicate higher purity). Overall,

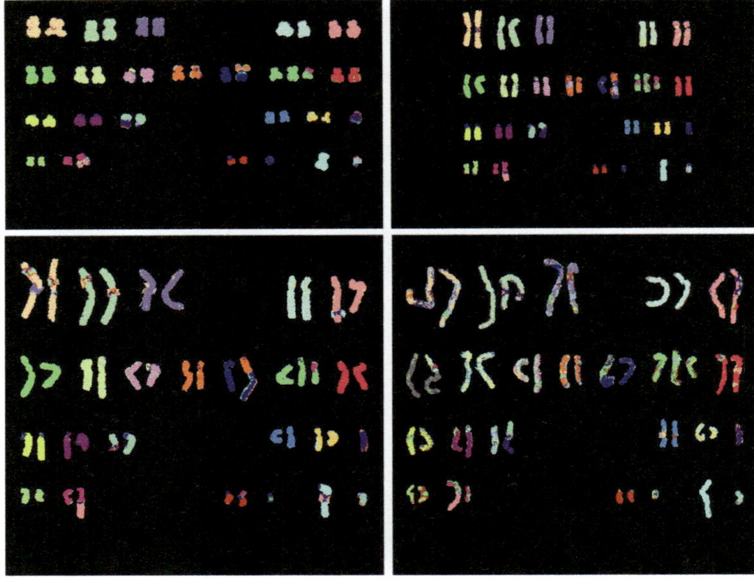

Fig. 9 Four color karyotypes for a single sample case with karyotype 45, XY, −18, −22, +11, t(7; 8), t(9; 10), t(11; 20), t(15; 18), t(20; 5)

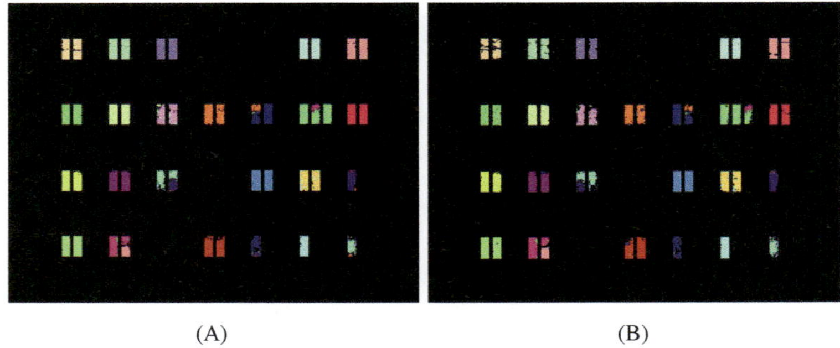

(A)   (B)

Fig. 10 (**A**) Prototype created by histogram-based. (**B**) Prototype created by eigen-based method

the performance of the eigen-based approach was lower with prototypes matching the ground-truth in 13 out of 15 cases. Moreover, the grouping efficiency was relatively low with only 8 cases showing 100 %. The eigen-based approach was more susceptible to color variability and out of 15 total cases tested, the histogram-based method outperformed eigenspace analysis in 7 cases with a smaller total variance within the groups. Figure 11 shows the comparison of total color variance between two methods for all the 15 cases.

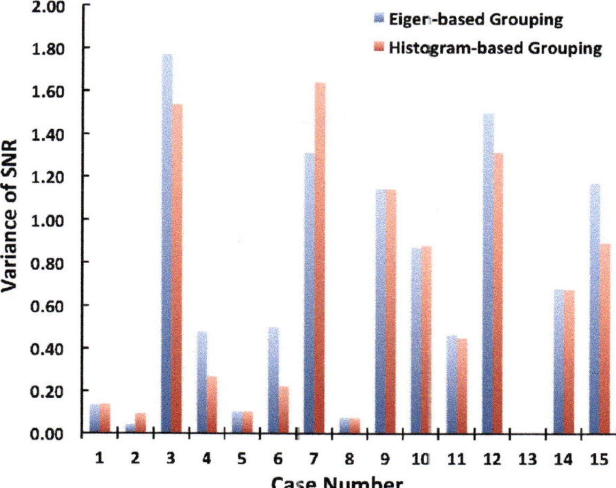

Fig. 11 Plot of color variance for the histogram and eigen-based chromosome grouping

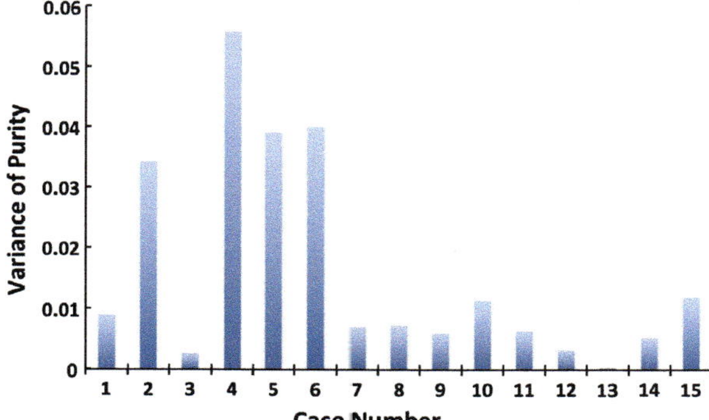

Fig. 12 Variability in color purity for the karyotypes analyzed

5 Conclusion

Color image analysis can be used to automatically generate representative proto-type karyotypes from a set of multiple karyotypes. The representative prototypes mirror aberrations from the multiple karyotypes while mitigating the appearance of misclassified pixels via color based pixel fusion. This allows a pictorial summary that depicts the aggregate information from multiple karyotypes thereby permitting convenient visualization and inference of any chromosomal aberrations. The statistical foundation of the chromosome grouping and fusion algorithms improves manual inference since overlapping chromosomes are resolved and misclassified pixels are automatically eliminated, whereas insertions and translocations are enhanced in the representative karyotype. Overall histogram based grouping not only provides an improved distance metric for clustering similar chromosomes, but also has an added advantage of reduced computational requirements when compared to the eigen-based approach. Further studies need to focus on automatically flagging the aberrations in the representative karyotypes while providing statistical confidence limits on the flagged aberrations.

References

1. Tjio JH, Levan A (1956) The chromosome number of man. Hereditas 42(1–2):1–6
2. Bayani JM, Squire JA (2002) Applications of SKY in cancer cytogenetics. Cancer Investig 20(3):373–386
3. Carpenter NJ (2001) Molecular cytogenetics. Semin Pediatr Neurol 8(3):135–146
4. Castleman KR, Melnyk J, Frieden HJ, Persinger GW, Wall RJ (1976) Karyotype analysis by computer and its application to mutagenicity testing of environmental chemicals. Mutat Res 41(1):153–161
5. Lee C, Lemyre E, Miron PM, Morton CC (2001) Multicolor fluorescence in situ hybridization in clinical cytogenetic diagnostics. Curr Opin Pediatr 13(6):550–555
6. Lundsteen C, Lind AM, Granum E (1976) Visual classification of banded human chromosomes. I. Karyotyping compared with classification of isolated chromosomes. Ann Hum Genet 40(1):87–97
7. Swansbury J (2003) Introduction to the analysis of the human G-banded karyotype. Methods Mol Biol 220:259–269
8. Todd R, Donoff RB, Wong DT (2000) The chromosome: cytogenetic analysis and its clinical application. J Oral Maxillofac Surg 58(9):1034–1039
9. Anderson R (2010) Multiplex fluorescence in situ hybridization (M-FISH). Methods Mol Biol 659:83–97
10. Speicher MR, Ward DC (1996) The coloring of cytogenetics. Nat Med 2(9):1046–1048
11. Liehr T, Starke H, Weise A, Lehrer H, Claussen U (2004) Multicolor FISH probe sets and their applications. Histol Histopathol 19(1):229–237
12. Schrock E, du Manoir S, Veldman T, Schoell B, Wienberg J, Ferguson-Smith MA, Ning Y, Ledbetter DH, Bar-Am I, Soenksen D, Garini Y, Ried T (1996) Multicolor spectral karyotyping of human chromosomes. Science 273(5274):494–497
13. Speicher MR, Gwyn Ballard S, Ward DC (1996) Karyotyping human chromosomes by combinatorial multi-fluor FISH. Nat Genet 12(4):368–375
14. Odero MD, Carlson K, Calasanz MJ, Lahortiga I, Chinwalla V, Rowley JD (2001) Identification of new translocations involving ETV6 in hematologic malignancies by fluorescence in situ hybridization and spectral karyotyping. Genes Chromosom Cancer 31(2):134–142
15. Castleman KR, Eils R, Morrison L, Piper J, Saracoglu K, Schulze MA, Speicher MR (2000) Classification accuracy in multiple color fluorescence imaging microscopy. Cytometry 41(2):139–147
16. Garini Y, Gil A, Bar-Am I, Cabib D, Katzir N (1999) Signal to noise analysis of multiple color fluorescence imaging microscopy. Cytometry 35(3):214–226
17. Rens W, Yang F, O'Brien PC, Solanky N, Ferguson-Smith MA (2001) A classification efficiency test of spectral karyotyping and multiplex fluorescence in situ hybridization: identification of chromosome homologies between homo sapiens and hylobates leucogenys. Genes Chromosom Cancer 31(1):65–74
18. Strefford JC, Lillington DM, Young BD, Oliver RT (2001) The use of multicolor fluorescence technologies in the characterization of prostate carcinoma cell lines: a comparison of multiplex fluorescence in situ hybridization and spectral karyotyping data. Cancer Genet Cytogenet 124(2):112–121
19. Lee C, Gisselsson D, Jin C, Nordgren A, Ferguson DO, Blennow E, Fletcher JA, Morton CC (2001) Limitations of chromosome classification by multicolor karyotyping. Am J Hum Genet 68(4):1043–1047

20. Azofeifa J, Fauth C, Kraus J, Maierhofer C, Langer S, Bolzer A, Reichman J, Schuffenhauer S, Speicher MR (2000) An optimized probe set for the detection of small interchromosomal aberrations by use of 24-color FISH. Am J Hum Genet 66(5):1684–1688
21. Jalal SM, Law ME (1999) Utility of multicolor fluorescent in situ hybridization in clinical cytogenetics. Genet Med 1(5):181–186
22. Knutsen T, Gobu V, Knaus R, Reid T, Sirotkin K (2002) The SKY/CGH database for spectral karyotyping and comparative genomic hybridization data. In: McEntyre J, Ostell J (eds) The NCBI handbook national center for biotechnology information, USA, Bethesda, MD
23. SD de Carvalho CR B (2003) A software tool to straighten curved chromosome images. Chromosom Res 11(1):83–88
24. Javan-Roshtkhari M, Setarehdan SK (2007) A new approach to automatic classification of the curved chromosomes. In: Proceedings of the 5th international symposium on image and signal processing and analysis, vol 1, pp 19–24
25. Choi HI, Choi SW, Moon HP (1997) Mathematical theory of medial axis transform. Pac J Math 181(1):57–88
26. Merchant FA, Good KN, Choi H, Castleman KR (2002) Automated detection of chromosomal rearrangements in multicolor fluorescence in-situ hybridization images. In: Proceedings of the second joint IEEE EMBS/BMES conference, vol 2, pp 1074–1075
27. Beran R (1977) Minimum Hellinger distance estimates for parametric models. Ann Stat 5(3):445–463
28. Sampat MP, Bovik AC, Aggarwal JK, Castleman KR (2005) Supervised parametric and non-parametric classification of chromosome images. Pattern Recognit 38(8):1209–1223
29. M-FISH chromosome imaging database (2012). http://live.ece.utexas.edu/research/mfish.html

Colour Model Analysis for Histopathology Image Processing

Gloria Bueno, Oscar Déniz, Jesús Salido, M. Milagro Fernández,
Noelia Vállez, and Marcial García-Rojo

Abstract This chapter presents a comparative study among different colour models (RGB, HSI, CMYK, CIEL*a*b*, and HSD) applied to very large microscopic image analysis. Such analysis of different colour models is needed in order to carry out a successful detection and therefore a classification of different regions of interest (ROIs) within the image. This, in turn, allows both distinguishing possible ROIs and retrieving their proper colour for further ROI analysis. This analysis is not commonly done in many biomedical applications that deal with colour images. Other important aspect is the computational cost of the different processing algorithms according to the colour model. This work takes these aspects into consideration to choose the best colour model tailored to the microscopic stain and tissue type under consideration and to obtain a successful processing of the histological image.

1 Introduction

Digitization in the biomedical field has become a reality thanks to the evolution of devices, applications. Anatomical Pathology has also benefited from these new technologies, which have provided solutions for whole slide scanning by means of motorized microscopes and scanners [14], that is, whole slide imaging (WSI). A WSI system equipped with the right storage and computing infrastructure can significantly improve workflow, hence increasing productivity while reducing costs, enable automated image analysis, quantification and quality control [8, 23, 26]. Ensuring optimal performance using the available technology depends essentially on the creation of computational tools that integrate mathematical and physical mod-

G. Bueno (✉) · O. Déniz · J. Salido · M. Milagro Fernández · N. Vállez
VISILAB, E.T.S.I.I, Universidad de Castilla-La Mancha, Avda. Camilo José Cela, 3,
13071 Ciudad Real, Spain
e-mail: gloria.bueno@uclm.es

M. García-Rojo
Dpt. Anatomía Patológica, Hospital General Universitario de Ciudad Real, C/ Obispo Rafael
Torija, s/n. 13005 Ciudad Real, Spain

M.E. Celebi, G. Schaefer (eds.), *Color Medical Image Analysis*,
Lecture Notes in Computational Vision and Biomechanics 6,
DOI 10.1007/978-94-007-5389-1_9, © Springer Science+Business Media Dordrecht 2013

els under defined architectures. The objective of this integration is to obtain and describe the necessary information for accurate interpretations in clinical diagnosis.

In this chapter we present a comparative study among different colour models (RGB, HSI, CMYK, CIEL*a*b*, and HSD). The colour models have been applied to very large microscopic image analysis. Such analysis of different colour models is needed in order to carry out a successful detection and therefore a classification of different regions of interest (ROIs) within the image. This, in turn, allows both distinguishing possible ROIs and retrieving their proper colour for further ROI analysis. This analysis is not commonly done in many biomedical applications that deal with colour images. Other important aspect is the computational cost of the different processing algorithms according to the colour model. This work takes these aspects into consideration to choose the best colour model tailored to the microscopic stain and tissue type under consideration and to obtain a successful processing of the histological image.

Several research works have sought to develop image processing algorithms for histological image analysis. Most of them are focused on the segmentation of only one region of interest (ROI), that is usually the nucleus and glands, as well as their classification for diagnosis purposes. To this end, Doyle et al. [12] use multi-resolution classification, first and second order statistics, as well as wavelet features, and support vector machines (SVM) for classification into benign and malign tissue. A multi-scale approach is also used in several works [18, 27, 32]. Huang et al. [18] use sparse coding and dynamic sampling where the computational time is reduced with GPU processing. Roullier et al. [32] and Madabhushi et al. [27] present graph-based multi-resolution approaches using domain specific knowledge. Other novel classification methods use neural networks [43], probability maps [10], and fractal dimension analysis [19].

Statistical information techniques [13], region growing algorithms [3, 29, 48], fuzzy c-means [2, 15, 28, 29] active contour models [17, 47], including level set methods [16, 44, 46], filtering and morphological analysis [3, 37, 40, 44] have been also used for ROI detection. The main problem with these methods is that they are not designed to process large amounts of data, which is the case when working with whole digital slides in pathology. The size of histological images may range from 300 Megabytes (MB) to 30 Gigabytes (GB) of RAW information, that is between 20000×20000 pixels to 100000×100000 pixels. However, usually only areas of a few Mbytes are processed, with the consequent risk of losing important information in the image. Thus, the image processing that slides are subject to is still limited both in terms of data processed and processing methods. Besides, many of these methods yield limited results because they focus mainly on a single structure or type of tissue.

Therefore, there is a need to design and develop parallel image processing tools for biomedical applications. To this end the colour model should be analysed, as well as the distance colour model applied to the processing algorithm in order to reduce the computational cost and obtain in an efficient way a set of heterogeneous, complex and specific image analysis. In this work different colour models and distances have been studied and applied under a general parallel image processing model designed and implemented with MPP (Massively Parallel Processing).

The evaluation of the colored stains at the specific subcellular regions where the markers are localized (i.e. nucleus, cellular membrane, cytoplasm) provides important information for the assessment of cancer [6, 41] Therefore, there are a few works in the literature to analyse and apply colour models for microscopic digital image processing. Van der Laak et al. [22] propose the HSD (Hue, Saturation, Density) model. The HSD model is an adaptation of the HSI model in which the RGB to HSI (Hue, Saturation, Intensity) transform is applied to optical densities (OD) for the individual RGB (Red, Green, Blue) channels instead of intensities. The use of OD has been also applied by Ruifrok et al. [33, 34] for quantification of immunohistochemical (IHC) staining. Thus they developed an algorithm to deconvolve the color information acquired with RGB cameras, to calculate the contribution of each of the applied stains, based on the stain-specific RGB absorption. This deconvolution method has been used to detect Ki-67 hot-spots on immunohistochemical slides of glioblastomas and separate the positive nuclei (brown) from the negative ones (blue) [25]. The deconvolution method has been also used combined with morphological methods for the segmentation of IHC tissue images of lung cancer [6, 7]. Recently, colour deconvolution was also used to assess the effect of potential therapeutic agents in dystrophic mice [31] and for quantitative image analysis of estrogen receptor, progesterone receptor, and Ki-67 IHC in breast cancer tissue sections [42].

The use of other colour models have been reported, mainly HSI and CMYK. Ficarra et al. use the HSI model to detect the membrane in non-small cell lung carcinoma IHC images and quantify the expression of growth factor receptor EGFR/erb-B family. HSI colour model is also used to help breast cancer diagnosis on breast tissue specimens stained separately for estrogen receptor, progesterone receptor and human epidermal growth factor receptor-2 (HER-2/neu) [30]. Other studies have been reported using HSI model to characterize medial fibrosis in relation to cardiovascular risk factors on TMA (tissue microarrays) [36]. A similar colour model, the HSL (Hue, Saturation, Luminance), has been used to quantify different IHC markers targeting proteins with different expression patterns (cytoplasmic, nuclear or membranous) in colon cancer or brain tumor TMAs [9].

2 Methods and Materials

2.1 Material Preparation

Tissue samples from biopsies and cytologies, prepared with different stains, were digitized with a motorized microscope ALIAS II at 20× with no compression. The samples were extracted from 8 lung cytologies and 8 prostate biopsies, with the diagnosis of carcinoma. Specimens fixed in 4 % buffered formalin were selected to prepare 4 mm thickness histological slides deparaffinized in xylene. Both conventional haematoxylin-eosin stain (HE) and immunohistochemical (IHQ) techniques were performed. In cytology Pap stain (Papanicolau) was performed. In all tissue cases, target retrieval was performed with a pre-treatment module for tissue specimens, PT Link, (DAKO, Denmark). Ready to use primary antibodies were incubated for 1 hour at room temperature, the detection was performed using the EnVision FLEX+ (DAKO, Denmark) visualization system in an Autostainer Link 48 (DAKO, Denmark).

Pap stain is a multichromatic staining cytological technique developed by George Papanikolaou. Pap staining is used to differentiate cells in smear preparations of various bodily secretions, here is used for pleural fluid. Pap staining is a very reliable technique. The classic form of Pap stain involves five dyes in three solutions [5]:

- A nuclear stain, haematoxylin, is used to stain cell nuclei. The unmordanted haematein may be responsible for the yellow color imparted to glycogen.
- First OG-6 counterstain (-6 denotes the used concentration of phosphotungstic acid; other variants are OG-5 and OG-8). Orange G is used. It stains keratin. Its original role was to stain the small cells of keratinizing squamous cell carcinoma present in sputum.
- Second EA (Eosin Azure) counterstain, comprising three dyes; the number denotes the proportion of the dyes, e.g. EA-36, EA-50, EA-65.
  - Eosin Y stains the superficial epithelial squamous cells, nucleoli, cilia, and red blood cells.
  - Light Green SF yellowish stains the cytoplasm of other cells, including non-keratinized squamous cells. This dye is now quite expensive and difficult to obtain, therefore some manufacturers are switching to Fast Green FCF, however it produces visually different results and is not considered satisfactory by some.
  - Bismarck brown Y stains nothing and in contemporary formulations it is often omitted.

When performed properly, the stained specimen should display hues from the entire spectrum: red, orange, yellow, green, blue, and violet. The chromatin patterns are well visible, the cells from borderline lesions are easier to interpret and the photomicrographs are better. The staining results in very transparent cells, so even thicker specimens with overlapping cells can be interpreted. On a well prepared specimen, the cell nuclei are crisp blue to black. Cells with high content of keratin are yellow, glycogen stains yellow as well. Superficial cells are orange to pink, and intermediate and parabasal cells are turquoise green to blue. Metaplastic cells often stain both green and pink at once. Pap stain is not fully standardized; it comes in several versions, subtly differing in the exact dyes used, their ratios, and timing of the process.

HE is a popular staining method in histology [1]. It is the most widely used stain in medical diagnosis; for example when a pathologist looks at a biopsy of a suspected cancer, the histological section is likely to be stained with HE section. The staining method involves application of hemalum, which is a complex formed from aluminium ions and oxidized haematoxylin. This colors nuclei of cells (and a few other objects, such as keratohyalin granules) blue. The nuclear staining is followed by counterstaining with an aqueous or alcoholic solution of eosin Y, which

Fig. 1 Two samples of histopathological images acquired at 20×

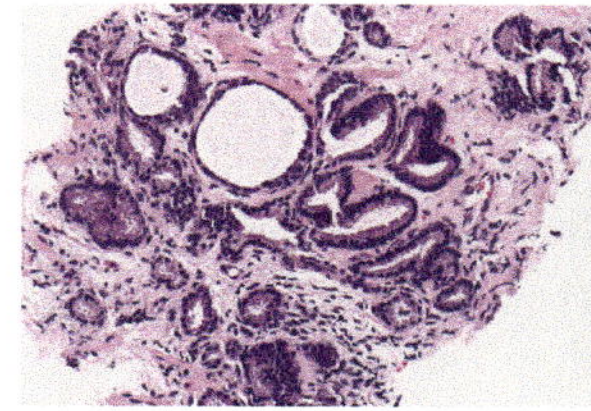

(a) Biopsy image

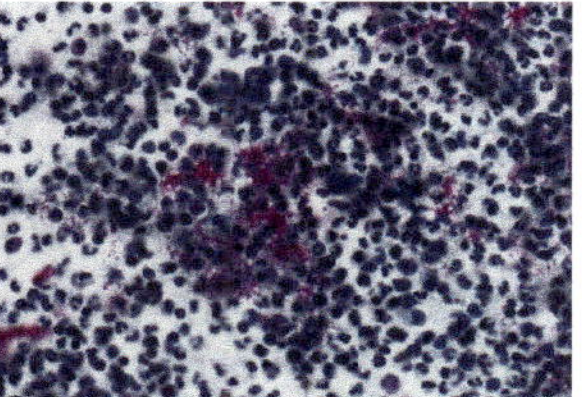

(b) Citology image

colors other, eosinophilic structures in various shades of red, pink and orange. The staining of nuclei by hemalum does not require the presence of DNA and is probably due to binding of the dye-metal complex to arginine-rich basic nucleoproteins such as histones. The mechanism is different from that of nuclear staining by basic (cationic) dyes such as thionine or toluidine blue. Staining by basic dyes is prevented by chemical or enzymatic extraction of nucleic acids. The eosinophilic structures are generally composed of intracellular or extracellular protein. Most of the cytoplasm is eosinophilic. Red blood cells are stained intensely red. Other colors, e.g. yellow and brown, can be present in the sample; they are caused by intrinsic pigments, e.g. melanin [21, 24].

The processing was done using our own libraries, implemented by the research group, running under MPI on a grid composed by 17 nodes Intel Xeon (3.2 GHz) INFINIBAND net (10 GB full-duplex) architecture. Two samples of the histopathological images analyzed are illustrated in Fig. 1.

2.2 Methods

This chapter compares five different colour models: RGB, HSI, CMYK, CIEL*a*b*, and HSD applied to histological WSI processing. Since these colour models are the most commonly used in histopathological image processing.

2.2.1 RGB Colour Model

The RGB colour model stands for the three additive primary colours, red, green, and blue. The main purpose of the RGB colour model is for the sensing, representation, and display of images in electronic systems, such as televisions and computers, though it has also been used in conventional photography. The RGB colour model has a solid theory based on human perception of colours, that is trichromacy. The normal explanation of trichromacy is that the organism's retina contains three types of colour receptors with different absorption spectra. The RGB colour model is based on the Young-Helmholtz theory of trichromatic colour vision, developed by Thomas Young and Hermann Helmholtz, in the early to mid nineteenth century, and on James Clerk Maxwell's colour triangle that elaborated that theory. Physiological evidence for trichromatic theory was later given by Gunnar Svaetichin (1956) [39].

The normal three kinds of light-sensitive photoreceptor cells in the human eye (cone cells) respond most to yellow (long wavelength or L), green (medium or M), and violet (short or S) light (peak wavelengths near 570 nm, 540 nm and 440 nm, respectively [20]. The difference in the signals received from the three kinds allows the brain to differentiate a wide gamut of different colours, while being most sensitive to yellowish-green light and to differences between hues in the green-to-orange region. During digital image processing each pixel can be represented in the computer memory or interface hardware (for example, a graphics card) as binary values for the red, green, and blue colour components. When properly managed, these values are converted into intensities or voltages via gamma correction to correct the inherent nonlinearity of some devices, such that the intended intensities are reproduced on the display.

The RGB colour model is the most common way to encode colour in computing, and several different binary digital representations are in use. Since colours are usually defined by three components, then a three-dimensional volume is described by treating the component values as Cartesian coordinates in a Euclidean space. For the RGB model, this is represented by a cube using non-negative values within a 0-1 range, assigning black to the origin (0, 0, 0), and with increasing intensity values running along the three axes up to white (1, 1, 1). An RGB triplet (r, g, b) represents the three-dimensional coordinate of the point of the given colour within the cube or its faces or along its edges. This approach allows computations of the colour similarity of two given RGB colours by simply calculating the distance between them: the shorter the distance, the higher the similarity.

2.2.2 HSI Colour Model

HSI stands for hue, saturation, and intensity. Other similar models are HSV where V stands for value, and is also often called HSB (B for brightness) and HSL where L stands for lightness. These colour models are the most common cylindrical-coordinate representations of points in an RGB colour model, which rearrange the geometry of RGB in an attempt to be more intuitive and perceptually relevant than the Cartesian (cube) representation. They were developed in the 1970s for computer graphics applications, in colour-modification tools in image editing software, and for image analysis and computer vision.

In each cylinder, the angle around the central vertical axis corresponds to hue, the distance from the axis corresponds to saturation, and the distance along the axis corresponds to intensity, lightness, value or brightness. Hue refers to the same attribute, while the definitions of saturation may differ. Because HSI is transformation of device-dependent RGB models, the physical colours they define depend on the colours of the red, green, and blue primaries of the device or of the particular RGB space, and on the gamma correction used to represent the amounts of those primaries. The resulting mixtures in RGB colour space can reproduce a wide variety of colours (called a gamut); however, the relationship between the constituent amounts of red, green, and blue light and the resulting colour is unintuitive. Furthermore, neither additive nor subtractive colour models define colour relationships the same way the human eye does [4, 11, 35]. In an attempt to accommodate more traditional and intuitive colour mixing models, the HSV model was developed in the mid-1970s [38]. The following year, 1979, at SIGGRAPH, Tektronix introduced graphics terminals using HSL for colour designation, and the Computer Graphics Standards Committee recommended it in their annual status report. These models were useful not only because they were more intuitive than raw RGB values, but also because the conversions to and from RGB were extremely fast to compute: they could run in real time on the hardware of the 1970s.

The drawback of these models is that they do not separate colour-making attributes, or their lack of perceptual uniformity. Perceptual uniformity means that a change of the same amount in a color value should produce a change of about the same visual importance. HSI, HSV and HSB colour models ignore much of the complexity of colour appearance. Other more computationally intensive models, such as CIEL*a*b* better achieve these goals. If we plot the RGB gamut in a more perceptually-uniform space, such as CIEL*a*b*, it becomes immediately clear that the red, green, and blue primaries do not have the same lightness or chroma, or evenly spaced hues.

2.2.3 CMYK Colour Model

The CMYK colour model (process colour, four colour) is a subtractive colour model, used in colour printing, and is also used to describe the printing process itself. CMYK refers to the four inks used in some colour printing: cyan, magenta, yellow, and key (black). Though it varies by print house, press operator, press manufacturer and press run, ink is typically applied in the order of the abbreviation. The "K" in CMYK stands for key since in four-colour printing cyan, magenta, and yellow printing plates are carefully keyed or aligned with the key of the black key plate.

The CMYK model works by partially or entirely masking colours on a lighter, usually white, background. The ink reduces the light that would otherwise be reflected. Such a model is called subtractive because inks "subtract" brightness from white. In the CMYK model, white is the natural colour of the paper or other background, while black results from a full combination of coloured inks. This is the opposite of additive colour models such as RGB, where white is the additive combination of all primary coloured lights, while black is the absence of light. However, both RGB and CMYK spaces, model the output of physical devices rather than human visual perception.

2.2.4 CIEL*a*b* Colour Model

The three coordinates of CIEL*a*b* represent the lightness of the colour ($L* = 0$ yields black and $L* = 100$ indicates diffuse white; specular white may be higher), its position between red/magenta and green ($a*$, negative values indicate green while positive values indicate magenta) and its position between yellow and blue ($b*$, negative values indicate blue and positive values indicate yellow). The CIEL*a*b* colour space is based on the CIEXYZ colour space coordinates. The CIEXYZ colour space simulate the perceived brightness by the human eyes, that is with sensitivity peaks in short (S, 420–440 nm), middle (M, 530–540 nm), and long (L, 560–580 nm) wavelengths. Y means brightness, Z is quasi-equal to blue stimulation, and X is a mix which looks like red sensitivity curve of cones. Thus, CIEL*a*b* colour model can predict which spectral power distributions will be perceived as the same colour (metamerism), but which is not particularly perceptually uniform. This property can improve the reproduction of tones.

The CIEL*a*b* colour space includes all perceivable colours which means that its gamut exceeds those of the RGB and CMYK colour models. CIEL*a*b* space is much larger than the gamut of computer displays, printers, or even human vision, a bitmap image represented as CIEL*a*b* requires more data per pixel to obtain the same precision as an RGB or CMYK bitmap. One of the most important attributes of the CIEL*a*b* model is the device independency. This means that the colours are defined independent of their nature of creation or the device they are displayed on. Therefore, it is used as an interchange format between different devices. CIEL*a*b* colour is designed to approximate human vision, and its L component closely matches human perception of lightness. It can thus be used to make accurate colour balance corrections by modifying any of the CIEL*a*b* components.

2.2.5 HSD Colour Model

HSD stands for hue, saturation, and density. The HSD transform was defined as the RGB to HSI transform applied to optical density (OD) values rather than intensities for the individual RGB channels [22]. The OD for a channel depends linearly on the amount of stain, given the absorption value of the stain at each channel, thus following Lambert-Beers' law of absorption. The overall measure for the OD can be defined as the average of the OD for the three channels. According to van der Laak et al. [22] a colour model used for recognition of stains in transmitted light microscopy should not be based on the human visual system. Instead, it should provide chromatic information independent of the OD of the stain. Thus, the HSD model should be suitable for stain recognition in digital images from transmitted light microscopy and enable all possible distinctions in a 2D standardised data space [22].

It is out of the scope of this chapter go deeply to the formulation to convert from the RGB colour model to others. The reader interested may refer to the cited bibliography [45].

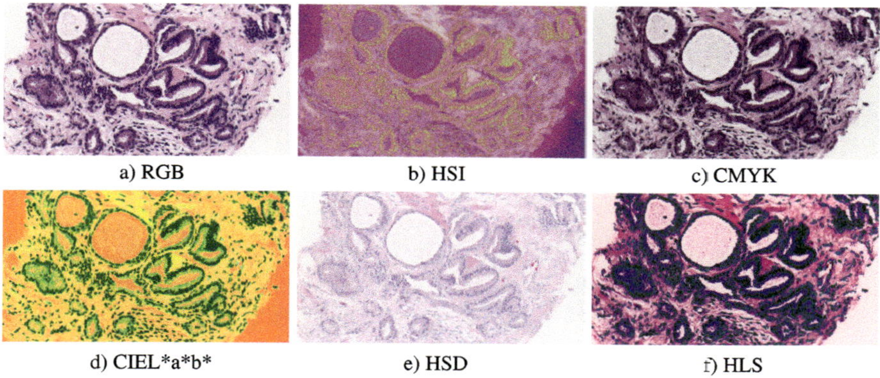

a) RGB   b) HSI   c) CMYK

d) CIEL*a*b*   e) HSD   f) HLS

Fig. 2 Colour models for the biopsy tissue sample

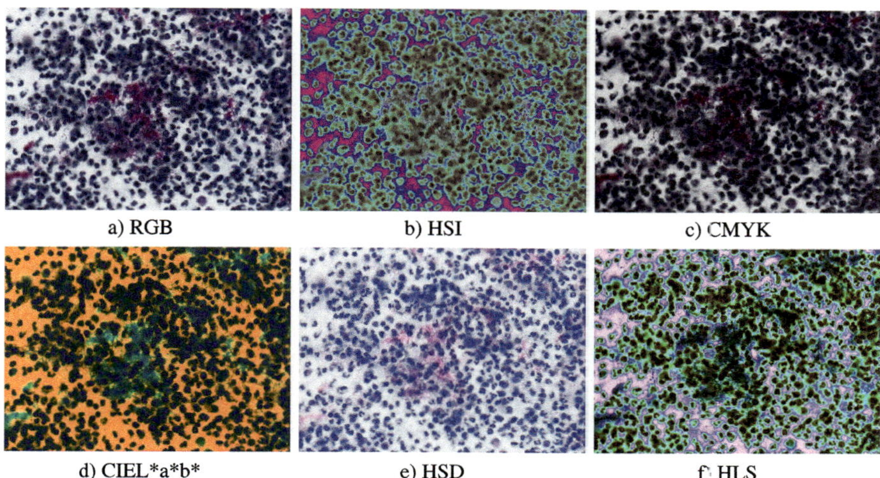

a) RGB   b) HSI   c) CMYK

d) CIEL*a*b*   e) HSD   f) HLS

Fig. 3 Colour models for the cytology tissue sample

Figures 2 and 3 show the different colour models for the biopsy and cytology tissue samples, respectively. Figure 4 shows all colour channels of the colour models for the biopsy tissue sample.

All colour models have their advantages and drawbacks. It is necessary to identify which colour model is suitable to represent and reproduce the ROI under consideration for each tissue type and WSI modality. This may be done by analysing the distance colour formulae applied between two colours, $d(\mathbf{x}, \mathbf{y})$, with $\mathbf{x} = (x_1, x_2, x_3)$ and $\mathbf{y} = (y_1, y_2, y_3)$.

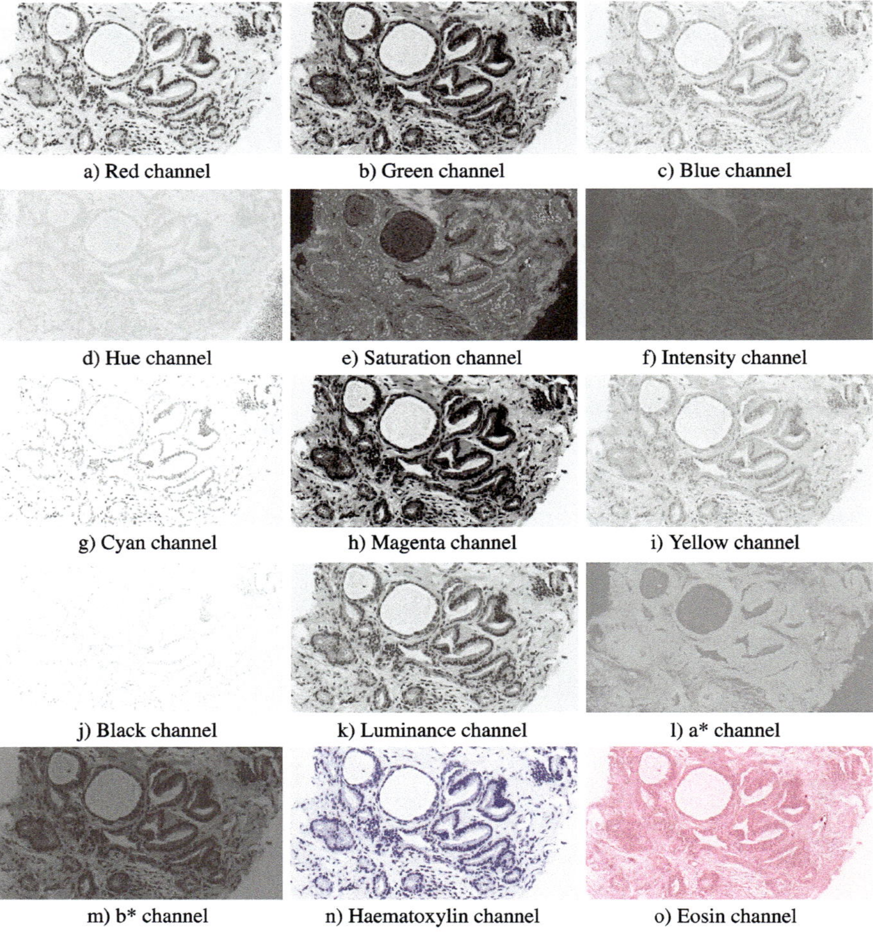

a) Red channel b) Green channel c) Blue channel

d) Hue channel e) Saturation channel f) Intensity channel

g) Cyan channel h) Magenta channel i) Yellow channel

j) Black channel k) Luminance channel l) a* channel

m) b* channel n) Haematoxylin channel o) Eosin channel

Fig. 4 Colour channels for the biopsy tissue sample

The distance considered within this study are: the Euclidean distance for the RGB model (see Eq. (1)), the NBS colour distance formulae for HSI model (see Eq. (2)) and the CIEDE2000 for the CIEL*a*b*, colour model (see Eq. (3)).

$$d(\mathbf{x}, \mathbf{y}) = \sqrt{(x_1 - y_1)^2 + (x_2 - y_2)^2 + (x_3 - y_3)^2} \tag{1}$$

$$d(\mathbf{x}, \mathbf{y}) = 1.2 * \sqrt{2x_2 y_2 \left(1 - \cos\left(\frac{2\pi \Delta H}{100}\right)\right) + \Delta S^2 + (4\Delta I)^2} \tag{2}$$

$$\Delta E_{00} = \sqrt{\left(\frac{\Delta L'}{K_L S_L}\right)^2 + \left(\frac{\Delta C'}{K_C S_C}\right)^2 + \left(\frac{\Delta H'}{K_H S_H}\right)^2 + R_T \left(\frac{\Delta C'}{K_C S_C}\right)\left(\frac{\Delta H'}{K_H S_H}\right)} \tag{3}$$

where K_L, K_c, K_H are weight factors and the rest of components, S_L, S_C, S_H, C', H', may be calculated by means of the, {L*, a*, b*} coordinates [45].

Moreover, another aspect to be considered is how to deal with the colour coordinates, that is as a vector or in a marginal way. These aspects have been analysed within this work. To this end the 3*2 distances to the most representative colour ROIs and statistically identified on the image were calculated on different WSI, that is to prostate biopsies and lung cytology stained with hematoxiline-eosine (HEO) and papanicolau. The results are shown as follows.

3 Results

The results applied to microscopic images show that the Euclidean and NBS vector distance for the RGB, HSI model respectively distinguish among different ROIs. The same occurs with the CMYK and HSD model. The vector CIEDE2000 distance for the CIEL*a*b* model reproduces in a better way the original colour. However, the computational cost of the last one is higher than the other colour models, about four times higher.

The first column of Figs. 5 and 6 show the segmentation into six classes of the biopsy and cytology tissue samples respectively. The classes represent the most relevant structures within the biopsy image. The classes were previously selected with their representative colour pixels. Then, the distance of each pixel to the six classes was calculated. Euclidean distance was used for the RGB and CMYK models, the NBS distance for the HSI and HSD models and the CIEDE2000 for the CIEL*a*b* model. The second column of Figs. 5 and 6 show the scatter plot of the segmented pixels for all the colour models. The scatter plots show that all distance formulae separate similarly the different classes. The worst results are obtained with the CMYK colour model.

To quantify the goodness of the distance formulae a ROC analysis was carried on for two of the classes corresponding to the lumen or glandular light and nucleus of the biopsy sample. The true pixels belonging to the ROIs were indicated by experts at Hospital General Universitario de Ciudad Real. Table 1 shows the ROC analysis for the Euclidean, NBS and CIEDE2000 colour distance applied to the RGB, HSI, CMYK, CIEL*a*b*, and HSD models for the biopsy tissue sample. It is shown that the % of specificity is higher for the CIEDE2000 distance with lower value of FP.

4 Conclusions

This chapter has presented a comparative study among RGB, HSI, CMYK, CIEL*a*b*, and HSD colour models applied to histological images. This analysis, in turn, allows both distinguishing possible regions of interest and retrieving their proper colour for further region analysis. The results applied to prostate biopsies stained with HE and lung cytologies stained with papanicolau show that the

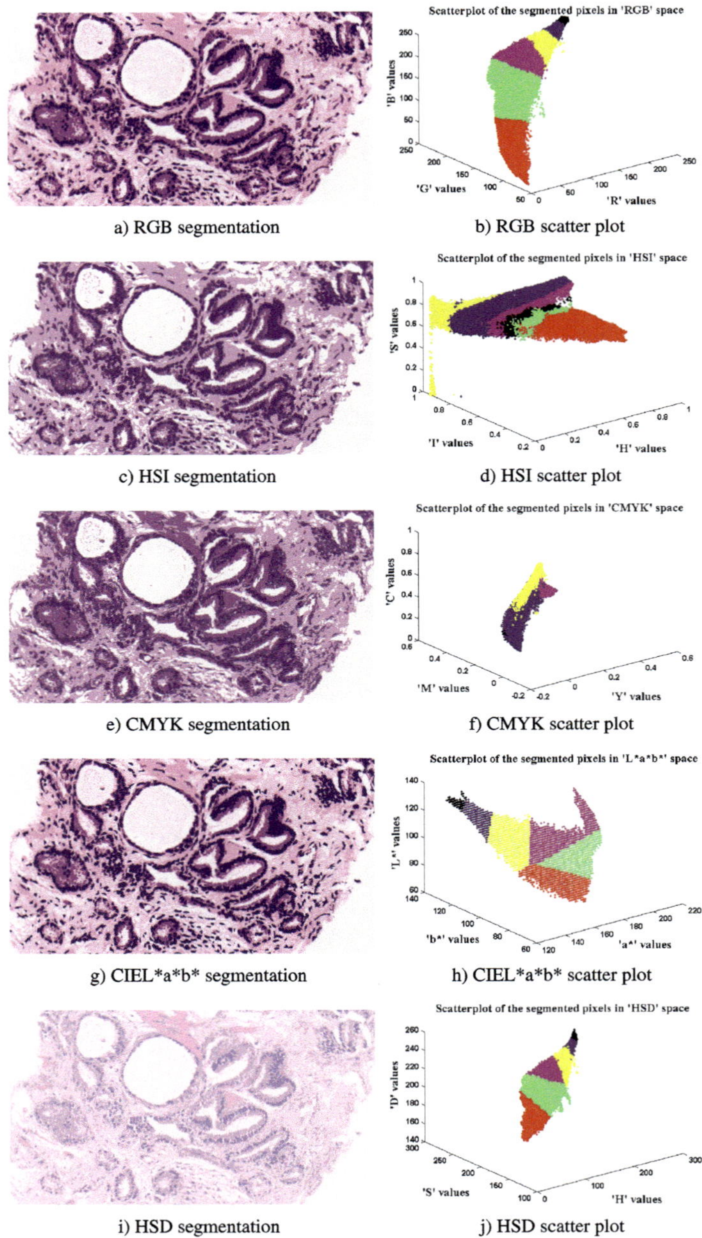

Fig. 5 Colour distance segmentation for the biopsy tissue sample

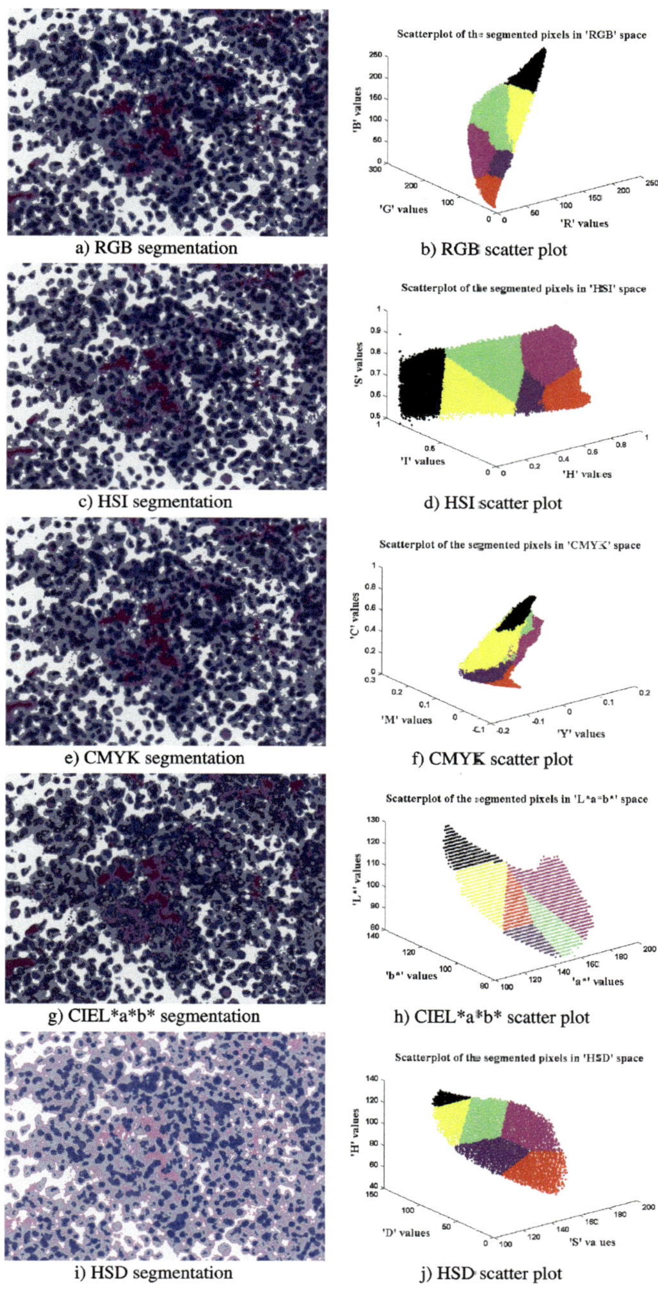

a) RGB segmentation   b) RGB scatter plot

c) HSI segmentation   d) HSI scatter plot

e) CMYK segmentation   f) CMYK scatter plot

g) CIEL*a*b* segmentation   h) CIEL*a*b* scatter plot

i) HSD segmentation   j) HSD scatter plot

Fig. 6 Colour distance segmentation for the cytology tissue sample

Table 1 ROC analysis of the colour distance formulae for the biopsy sample

(a) Glandular Light ROI

	FP	FN	TP	Specificity
RGB (Euclidean)	0.0165	0.0669	0.9330	0.9834
HSI (NBS)	0.0067	0.0900	0.9097	0.9932
CMYK (Euclidean)	0.0075	0.0703	0.8852	0.8827
CIEL*a*b* (CIEDE2000)	0.0047	0.1007	0.9082	0.9952
HSD (NBS)	0.0085	0.083	0.9417	0.9863

(b) Nucleus ROI

	FP	FN	TP	Specificity
RGB (Euclidean)	0.1542	0.0406	0.9593	0.8457
HSI (NBS)	0.0992	0.1090	0.8909	0.9007
CMYK (Euclidean)	0.0703	0.0427	0.9101	0.7591
CIEL*a*b* (CIEDE2000)	0.0573	0.2230	0.7717	0.9426
HSD (NBS)	0.0798	0.0507	0.9682	0.9128

vector CIEDE2000 distance for the CIEL*a*b* model reproduces in a better way the original colour.

Therefore, this comparison does allow us to choose the best colour model tailored to the microscopic stain and tissue type under consideration to obtain a successful processing. Moreover, a compromise between the computational cost and the results focus always to distinguish between different colour detection and colour retrieval for further ROI analysis should be kept. The colour model should be taken into consideration when defining standards for histological images.

Acknowledgements This work has been carried out with the support of the research projects DPI2008-06071 of the Spanish Research Ministry, PI-2010/040 of the FISCAM and PAI08-0283-9663 of JCCM. We extend our gratitude to the Department of Pathology at Hospital General Universitario de Ciudad Real for providing the tissue samples.

References

1. Avwioro G (2011) Histochemical uses of haematoxylin—a review. J Pharm Clin Sci 1:24–34
2. Begelman G, Gur E, Rivlin E, Rudzsky M, Zalevsky Z (2004) Cell nuclei segmentation using fuzzy logic engine. In: Proceedings of the IEEE international conference on image processing, pp 2937–2940
3. Belkacem-Boussaid K, Samsi S, Lozanski G, Gurcan MN (2011) Automatic detection of follicular regions in H&E images using iterative shape index. Comput Med Imaging Graph 35(7–8):592–602
4. Berk T, Kaufman A, Brownston L (1982) A human factors study of color notation systems for computer graphics. Commun ACM 25(8):547–550
5. Carson F, Hladik C (2009) Histotechnology: a self-instructional text, 3rd edn. American Society for Clinical Pathology, Hong Kong

6. Cataldo SD, Ficarra E, Acquaviva A, Macii E (2010) Achieving the way for automated segmentation of nuclei in cancer tissue images through morphology-based approach: a quantitative evaluation. Comput Med Imaging Graph 34(6):453–461

7. Cataldo SD, Ficarra E, Acquaviva A, Macii E (2010) Automated segmentation of tissue images for computerized IHC analysis. Comput Methods Programs Biomed 100(1):1–15

8. Daniel C, Rojo MG, Klossa J, Della Mea V, Booker D, Beckwith BA, Schrader T (2011) Standardizing the use of whole slide images in digital pathology. Comput Med Imaging Graph 35(7–8):496–505

9. Decaestecker C, Lopez XM, D'Haene N, Roland I, Guendouz S, Duponchelle C, Berton A, Debeir O, Salmon I (2009) Requirements for the valid quantification of immunostains on tissue microarray materials using image analysis. Proteomics 9(19):4478–4494

10. DiFranco MD, O'Hurley G, Kay EW, Watson, Cunningham P (2011) Ensemble based system for whole-slide prostate cancer probability mapping using color texture features. Comput Med Imaging Graph 35(7–8):629–645

11. Douglas S, Kirkpatrick A (1999) Model and representation: the effect of visual feedback on human performance in a color picker interface. ACM Trans Graph 18(2):96–127

12. Doyle S, Feldman M, Tomaszewski J, Madabhushi A (2012) A boosted bayesian multi-resolution classifier for prostate cancer detection from digitized needle biopsies. In: IEEE transactions on biomedical engineering, pp 1–14

13. Gao M, Bridgman P (2003) Computer aided prostate cancer diagnosis using image enhancement and JPEG2000. In: Proceedings of the SPIE international conference on applications of digital image processing, vol 5203, pp 323–334

14. García M, Bueno G, Peces C, González J, Carbajo M (2006) Critical comparison of 31 commercially available digital slide systems in pathology. Int J Surg Pathol 14(4):285–305

15. Hafiane A, Bunyak F, Palaniappan K (2008) Fuzzy clustering and active contours for histopathology image segmentation and nuclei detection. In: Advanced concepts for intelligent vision systems, vol 5259, pp 903–914

16. Hafiane A, Bunyak F, Palaniappan K (2008) Level set-based histology image segmentation with region-based comparison. In: Proceedings of the third international workshop on microscopic image analysis with applications in biology

17. Hu MP, Ding XY (2004) Automated cell nucleus segmentation using improved snake. In: Proceedings of the IEEE international conference on image processing, vol 4, pp 2737–2740

18. Huang CH, Veillard A, Roux L, Loménie N, Racoceanu D (2011) Time-efficient sparse analysis of histopathological whole slide images. Comput Med Imaging Graph 35:579–591

19. Huang PW, Lee CH (2009) Automatic classification for pathological prostate images based on fractal analysis. IEEE Trans Med Imaging 28(7):1037–1050

20. Hunt R (2004) The reproduction of colour, 6th edn. Wiley-IS&T series in imaging science and technology

21. Kiernan J (2008) Histological and histochemical methods: theory and practice, 4th edn. Scion Publishing Ltd, Bloxham

22. der Laak JV, Pahlplatz M, Hanselaar A, de Wilde P (2000) Hue-saturation-density (HSD) model for stain recognition in digital images from transmitted light microscopy. Cytometry 39(4):275–284

23. Lezoray O, Gurcan M, Can A, Olivo-Marin JC (2011) Whole slide microscopic image processing—special issue editorial. Comput Med Imaging Graph 35(7–8):493–495

24. Llewellyn B (2009) Nuclear staining with alum-hematoxylin. Biotech Histochem 84:159–177

25. Lopez XM, Debeir O, Maris C, Roland I, Salmon I, Decaestecker C (2010) KI-67 hot-spots detection on glioblastoma tissue sections, pp 149–152

26. Madabhushi A (2009) Digital pathology image analysis: opportunities and challenges. Imag Med 1(1):7–10

27. Madabhushi A, Agner S, Basavanhally A, Doyle S, Lee G (2011) Computer-aided prognosis: predicting patient and disease outcome via quantitative fusion of multi-scale, multi-modal data. Comput Med Imaging Graph 35(7–8):506–514

28. Naik S, Doyle S, Agner S, Madabhushi A, Feldman M, Tomaszewski J (2008) Automated gland and nuclei segmentation for grading of prostate and breast cancer histopathology. In: Proceedings of the 2008 IEEE international symposium on biomedical imaging: from nano to macro, pp 284–287
29. Peng Y, Jiang Y, Eisengart L, Healy M, Straus FH, Yang X (2011) Computer-aided identification of prostatic adenocarcinoma: segmentation of glandular structures. J Pathol Inform 2(33):1–10
30. Prasad K, Tiwari A, Ilanthodi S, Prabhu G, Pai M (2011) Automation of immunohistochemical evaluation in breast cancer using image analysis. World J Clin Oncol 2(4):187–194
31. van Putten M, de Winter C, van Roon-Mom W, van Ommen G, Hoen P, Aartsma-Rus A (2010) A 3 months mild functional test regime does not affect disease parameters in young mdx mice. Neuromuscul Disord 20:273–283
32. Roullier V, Lezoray O, Ta VT, Elmoataz A (2011) Multi-resolution graph-based analysis of histopathological whole slide images: application to mitotic cell extraction and visualization. Comput Med Imaging Graph 35(7–8):603–615
33. Ruifrok A, Johnston D (2001) Quantification of histological staining by color deconvolution. Anal Quant Cytol Histol 23:291–299
34. Ruifrok A, Katz R, Johnston D (2004) Comparison of quantification of histochemical staining by hue-saturation-intensity (HSI) transformation and color deconvolution. Appl Immunohistochem Mol Morphol 11(1):85–91
35. Schwarz M, Cowan W, Beatty J (1987) An experimental comparison of RGB, YIQ, LAB, HSV, and opponent color models. ACM Trans Graph 6(2):123–158
36. Selvin E, Najjar S, Cornish T, Halushka M (2010) A comprehensive histopathological evaluation of vascular medial fibrosis: insights into the pathophysiology of arterial stiffening. Atherosclerosis 208(1):69–74
37. Sertel O, Lozanski G, Shana'ah A, Gurcan MN (2010) Computer-aided detection of centroblasts for follicular lymphoma grading using adaptive likelihood-based cell segmentation. IEEE Trans Biomed Eng 57(10):2613–2616
38. Smith A (1982) Color gamut transform pairs. Comput Graph 12(3):12–19
39. Svaetichin G (1956) Spectral response curves from single cones. Actaphysiol 134:17–46
40. Tabesh A, Kumar V, Verbel D, Kotsianti A, Teverovskiy M, Saidi O (2002) Automated prostate cancer diagnosis and Gleason grading of tissue microarrays. In: Proceedings of the SPIE medical imaging conference, vol 5747, pp 58–70
41. Taneja T, Sharma S (2004) Markers of small cell lung cancer. World J Surg Oncol 2:10
42. Tuominen V, Ruotoistenmaki S, Viitanen A, Jumppanen M, Isola J (2010) ImmunoRatio: a publicly available web application for quantitative image analysis of estrogen receptor (ER), progesterone receptor (PR), and Ki-67. Breast Cancer Res 12(4):R56
43. Valenzuela O, Rojas I, Rojas F, Fernandez L (2005) Automatic classification of prostate cancer using pseudo-Gaussian radial basis function neural network. In: Proceedings of the European symposium on artificial neural networks, pp 145–150
44. Vidal J, Bueno G, Galeotti J, García-Rojo M, Relea F, Déniz O (2011) A fully automated approach to prostate biopsy segmentation based on level-set and mean filtering. J Pathol Inform 2(5):1–11
45. Wyszecki G, Stiles W (2000) Color science: concepts and methods, quantitative data and formulae, 2nd edn. Wiley, New York
46. Xu J, Madabhushi A, Janowczyk A, Chandran S (2010) A weighted mean shift, normalized cuts initialized color gradient based geodesic active contour model: applications to histopathology image segmentation. Proceedings of the SPIE medical imaging conference, vol 7623
47. Yang L, Meer P, Foran D (2005) Unsupervised segmentation based on robust estimation and colour active contour models. IEEE Trans Inf Technol Biomed 9(3):475–486
48. Yongming L, Dongming L, Xiqun L, Jianming L (2004) Interactive colour image segmentation by region growing combines with image enhancement based on Bezier model. In: Proceedings of the third international conference on image and graphics, vol 100, pp 96–99

A Review on CAD Tools for Burn Diagnosis

Aurora Sáez, Carmen Serrano, and Begoña Acha

Abstract A correct first treatment is essential for a favorable evolution of a burn injury. To know the depth of the burn is necessary to develop an appropriate course of treatment: correct visual assessment of burn depth relies highly on specialized dermatological expertise. The cost of maintaining a burn treatment unit is high, therefore it would be desirable to have an automatic system to give a first assessment at primary health-care centers, where there is a lack of specialists. The aim of the system is to separate burn wounds from healthy skin, and to distinguish among different types of burn depth. Digital color photographs are used as inputs to the system. Firstly, some topics related to image acquisition will be addressed. A method to normalize colors when photographs have been acquired with different cameras and/or illuminant conditions is described. Secondly, a comparative of several color segmentation algorithms will be presented. Finally, to estimate the burn depth a classification method, that take into account different color-texture features extracted from the burn images, will be described.

1 Introduction

For a favourable evolution of a burn injury, it is essential to initiate the correct first treatment [10]. To know the depth of the burn is necessary to develop an appropriate course of treatment: correct visual assessment of burn depth relies highly on specialized dermatological expertise. As the cost of maintaining a burn treatment unit is high, it would be desirable to have an objective or automatic system to give a first assessment at primary health-care centers, where there is a lack of specialists [32, 36]. The World Health Organization demands that, at least, there must be one

A. Sáez (✉) · C. Serrano · B. Acha
Dpto. Teoría de la señal y comunicaciones, E.T.S. de Ingeniería, Cmno. Descubrimientos s/n,
41092 Sevilla, Spain
e-mail: aurorasaez@us.es

C. Serrano
e-mail: cserrano@us.es

B. Acha
e-mail: bacha@us.es

M.E. Celebi, G. Schaefer (eds.), *Color Medical Image Analysis*,
Lecture Notes in Computational Vision and Biomechanics 6,
DOI 10.1007/978-94-007-5389-1_10, © Springer Science+Business Media Dordrecht 2013

bed in a Burn Unit for each 500,000 inhabitants. So, normally, one Burn Unit covers a large geographic area. If a burn patient appears in a medical centre without a Burn Unit, telephone communication is usually established between the closest hospital with a Burn Unit and the local medical centre, where the non-expert doctor describes subjectively the colour, size and other aspects considered important for burn characterization. The result in many cases is the application of an incorrect first treatment (very important, on the other hand, for a correct outcome for the patient and the wound), or unnecessary transportation of the patient, involving high Healthcare cost and psychological trauma for patients and family [30].

Procedures and systems for computer-aided diagnosis (CAD) [12, 13, 29] have gained increasing acceptance in medicine. However, the extension of the CAD concept to the analysis of color images of skin lesions is being developing at a slower pace due to difficulties in translating human color perception into objective rules that may be analyzed by a computer.

Automatic burn wound diagnosis is still a unexplored field. In the related bibliography, it can found that there is a tendency to investigate objective methods for determining the depth of the burn in order to reduce the subjectivity and the high experience requirement that visual inspection demands. In this sense, there are works trying to evaluate burn depth by using thermographic images [11, 33, 34], terahertz pulsed imaging [19], polarization-sensitive optical coherence tomography [27] and laser Doppler imaging [23, 24]. Afromowitz et al. [4, 5] try to give a diagnosis of the burn depth from a estimation of the number of days that the wound will take to heal. They measure the optic reflectivity in the red, green and infrared bands, hypothesizing that it is highly correlated with burn healing time, and they form a false colour image that indicates the time of healing, or equivalently, the depth of the burn. Renkielska et al. [31] present active dynamic thermography (ADT) as a quantitative method for burn wound discrimination by evaluating the thermal time constants. The main disadvantage of these methods is the complexity and cost of the image acquisition system.

Roa et al. [32] proposed the use of a digital photographic camera to develop an affordable image-acquisition method that met the following clinical needs:

- The system should not be expensive because the cost involved in a realistic implementation of the system should be low.
- The system should be easy to use by a physician or nurse because technicians specialized in acquiring images will not be usually available at primary medical centers.
- The system should preserve the essential characteristics of the burn wounds required for diagnosis.

In this sense, the group of Acha and Serrano [3, 37] has designed a clinically feasible system for automatic burn wound classification based on visual digital images. To achieve this aim, the following tasks have to be performed:

- Clinical needs establishment and development of the image acquisition protocol.
- *Digital image processing*: Once the image is acquired following a standardized protocol, it is processed to get the information required for assessing the burn

depth. Image-processing algorithms to isolate the burn from the rest of the scene (segmentation), and to give the depth of the segmented burn part (classification) have been designed.

- *System validation*: The system has been validated by a group of experts of a Burn Unit.

In this chapter a review of CAD system for burns diagnosis in digital color photographs is presented. This involves some topics related to image acquisition and color images characterization, color segmentation algorithms to isolate the burn wound from the rest of the scene and methods to estimate the burn depth.

2 Color Image Acquisition

All the research efforts published in the literature go in the line of finding new acquisition methods to analyse the depth of the burn [11, 19, 33, 34]. This is motivated by the fact that the diagnosis by simple inspection is difficult even for an expert doctor. Nevertheless, efforts described in this chapter have the color photograph as acquisition method. Therefore in this Section, methods to maintain image independent from the acquisition condition are analysed.

One of the main characteristics in the assessment of a burn wound that physicians take into account is color; therefore, an image-acquisition system must preserve this property to the highest accuracy possible.

Roa et al. [32] proposed a digital photographic camera as image acquisition device, which has a low cost and it is easy to use, essential for primary medical centers.

The main problem encountered in the analysis of digital photographs of burn wounds is that, in practical situations, the illumination conditions in hospitals are uncontrolled. As a result, the measured pixel values depend on the illuminants; with multiple illuminants, the measured values cannot be accurately converted to a known color space without additional information.

In the works of Serrano et al. [38] and Sáez et al. [35], two issues are discussed:

1. Experiments to study the influence of the most common illuminants encountered in hospitals. As a result, it is shown that the xenon flash dominates the ambient illumination. This is an important issue because the users will need to apply the characterization method only for each camera and not each time the illumination conditions change.
2. A colorimetric characterization algorithm that allows to convert RGB values under unknown illuminant to RGB values under D50 illuminant.

2.1 *Influence of Different Illumination Conditions*

In the study conducted by Serrano et al. [38], images of the Macbeth Color Checker® DC (Gretag-Macbeth GmbH, Martinsried, Germany) were acquired un-

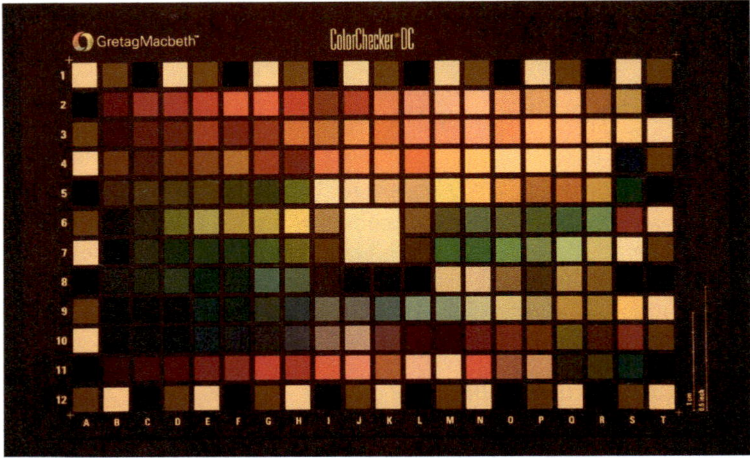

Fig. 1 The Macbeth Color Checker® chart DC (Gretag-Macbeth GmbH, Martinsried, Germany) captured under halogen illuminant

der carefully controlled conditions in order to separate out the various factors affecting the process. The images were captured in a dark room where all ambient light could be excluded, and therefore, an image under a unique illumination source could be taken (xenon flash, halogen or fluorescent light). Also, to take into account the possibility of natural illumination, images were acquired outdoors in diffuse sunlight. See Fig. 1 for illustration of an image of the Macbeth Color Checker® chart obtained under halogen illuminant.

The experiment was performed with a Digital Reflex Canon EOS 300D camera (Canon Inc., Tokyo, Japan), but the system was designed to be used with any type of digital camera. The distance between the camera and the object was fixed at approximately 0.5 m. A xenon flash was included in the camera. The positions of the fluorescent lamps in the ceiling were not specified. The camera aperture (Av) and focus were fixed at specific positions. In order to analyze the influence of different illuminants, the exposure time (Tv) was varied. An exposure time was considered to be optimal under a particular illuminant when it was at the maximum possible value without saturating any channel. The ratio between the exposure times gives an indication of the influence of the different sources of light. The optimal exposure times obtained were $Tv = 1/200$ s, 0.6 s, and 1.6 s with the xenon flash, sunlight, and fluorescent light, respectively. The exposure times indicate that the flash is 320 times stronger than the fluorescent light used and 120 times stronger than the sunlight conditions in the experiments. In other words, if $Tv = 1/200$ s and 8 bits are used per color component, the fluorescent light will not influence even the least significant bit (LSB); the sunlight conditions will influence two LSBs. In another analysis, the maximal pixel values obtained under flash illumination, under daylight plus fluorescent illumination, and with no illu-

Table 1 Maximal pixel values of a photograph of the Macbeth Color Checker® DC (Gretag-Macbeth GmbH, Martinsried, Germany) for different illumination conditions with the same camera parameters

Illumination	R	G	B
Flash	227	196	188
Fluorescent light and sunlight	5	7	4
No illumination	4	5	4

mination at all (with the lens of the camera covered with its cap) were compared. The same camera parameters ($Av = 20$, $ISO = 100$, $Tv = 1/200$ s) were used. Taking a photograph under both the fluorescent and sunlight illumination conditions with $Tv = 1/200$ s would yield images with only two LSBs having nonzero values.

The results, summarized in Table 1, confirm that all of the illumination conditions evaluated other than the xenon flash influence only the two LSBs.

Therefore, Acha et al. in [3] proposed the following acquisition protocol for burn wounds: distance between camera and patient should be about 40–50 cm, the background should be a green/blue sheet, the flash must be on and the camera should be placed parallel to the burn wound. The parameters of the camera were set to: ISO speed 100, exposure time 1/200 s and aperture (f stop) 20.

2.2 Colorimetric Characterization Algorithm

An additional problem encountered is the camera cannot perform the chromatic adaptation that the human eye automatically performs. Therefore, a photographed surface with several illuminants show different colors for each illuminant. In [35] is proposed a characterization method based on the Gretag-Macbeth Color Checker target [39]. The authors used the Macbeth ColorChecker DC chart with 240 color chips. It is supplied with data giving the CIE XYZ chromaticity coordinates of each chip under D50 illuminant. The algorithm creates interpolation curves using spline cubic interpolation, based on points formed by RGB values of gray chips of the photographed chart under unknown illuminat and the RGB values for these gray chips, under D50 illuminat, provided by the manufacturer. These interpolation curves are applied to the photographed images under the same unknown illuminant that Macbeth ColorChecker DC chart was captured. The RGB values of these images under the unknown illuminant are matched with RGB values under D50 illuminant.

In order to illustrate the performance of the algorithm, a magenta color sheet was photographed under four different illuminants: a halogen lamp, fluorescent lights, a xenon flash, and afternoon sunlight. Figure 2 shows the photographs obtained under the different illuminants before and after the characterization step. It can be

Fig. 2 A magenta sheet photographed under four different illumination conditions: (**a**) a xenon flash, (**b**) afternoon sunlight, (**c**) fluorescent lights, and (**d**) a halogen lamp. (**e**)–(**h**) The characterized images corresponding to the images in (**a**)–(**d**), respectively

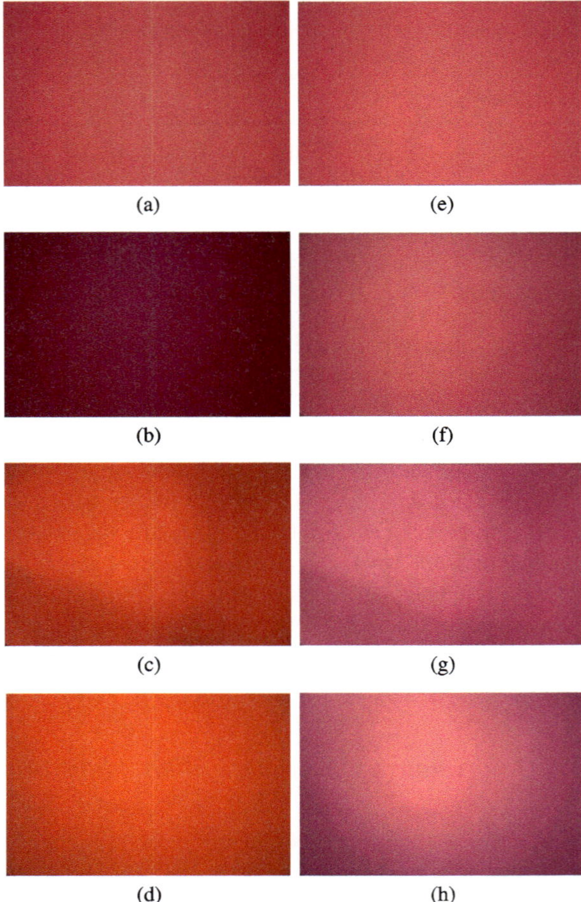

observed that, after the characterization procedure, the four photographs present similar colors.

3 Segmentation

Different segmentation methods have been applied in the literature to segment burn wounds. In her PhD thesis [1], Acha proposed a segmentation method based on color analysis. It was applied to a small database. Result images were presented but a quantitative analysis of the segmentation is missing. In [3] a new method is presented and a quantitative evaluation, with comparison to manual segmentation, is shown. Finally, Castro et al. [9] present results of the segmentation of burns with different fuzzy-cmeans algorithms. In the following subsections, the former algorithms will be described and results for each of them will be presented.

3.1 Segmentation Based on Angular Distances Applied to Hue

In this algorithm [1] burn images are segmented following the steps described below.

Preprocessing. In this preprocessing step the image is transform to hue, saturation and lightness (L^*) according to the transform standardized by CIE in 1976 [22]. Then, an anisotropic diffusion is applied to the chromatic and achromatic information [21, 26].

Image transform to a one-channel image. Through a color analysis, the color image is transformed to a one-plane image where the burn is in the most left side of the histogram. To this aim a minimum intervention of the user is required: a point inside the burn must be selected with the mouse. This will be considered the burn color, $(L_b^*, h_{uvb}, s_{uvb})$. The objective of this step is to transform the color information of each pixel in the image, (L^*, h_{uv}, s_{uv}), described by means of hue and saturation, into an only parameter, d_{uv}, correlated to the color difference between each pixel in the image and the pixel selected by the user inside the burn. This parameter must be low inside the burn and higher in the rest of the image. Thus color differences to the selected point could be used. In this algorithm, a combination of an angular distance for the hue and linear distance for the saturation was proposed. In particular, the distance between h_{uv} and h_{uvb} was estimated with an expression similar to the Von Mises distribution of the difference of both quantities as:

$$d_{uvh}(n, m) = \frac{h_{uvb}}{\exp(W)} \exp\left(W \cos\left(h_{uv}(n, m) - h_{uvb}\right)\right), \tag{1}$$

where W is the parameter that controls the selectivity around h_{uvb} of the function $d_{uv}(n, m)$. As regards to saturation, in [1] the distance between s_{uv} and s_{uvb} is modelled as the Gaussian of the scalar difference:

$$d_{uvs}(n, m) = s_{uvb} \exp\left(-\frac{(s_{uv}(n, m) - s_{uvb})^2}{2\sigma_c^2}\right), \tag{2}$$

where σ_c controls the selectivity of the function d_{uvs}. W and σ_c were fixed experimentally, equal for all the database, according to the variability that hue and saturation present within each burn wound. Finally d_{uvh} and d_{uvs} were combined as:

$$d_{uv} = \beta d_{uvh} + (1 - \beta)d_{uvs} \tag{3}$$

According to [1], the weight β is a parameter that varies between 0 and 1 and weights the importance of hue or saturation in the burn perception. Segmentation results for some images from the database are presented in Figs. 3, 4 and 5. They are shown in comparison to segmentation obtained with the algorithm presented in [3], explained below.

3.2 Segmentation Based on Color Distances

The segmentation approach used here is a supervised pixel-based algorithm based on measures in the CIE L*u*v* color coordinate space. L*u*v* and L*a*b* color

Fig. 3 Segmentation results:
(**a**) Original image,
(**b**) Segmentation based on
angular distances applied to
hue, (**c**) Segmentation based
on color distances

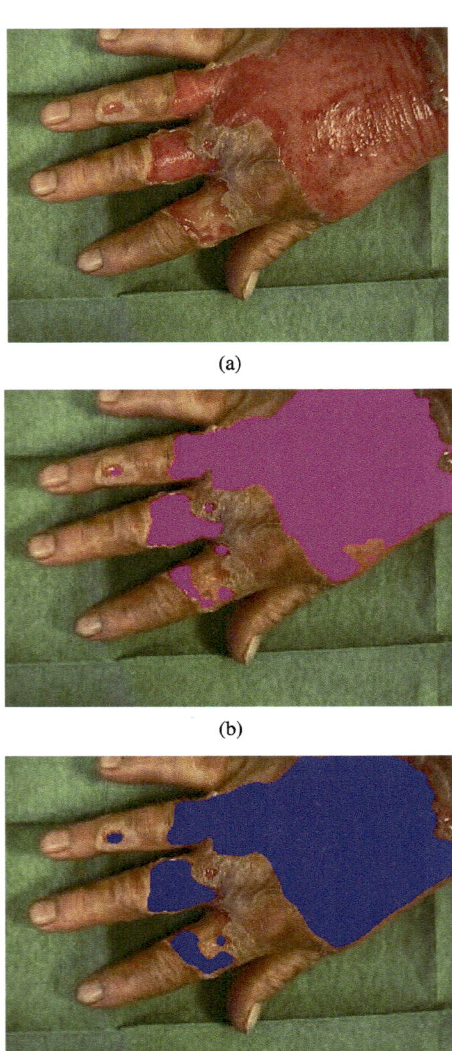

(a)

(b)

(c)

representation systems are called uniform systems because Euclidean distances between colors measured in these spaces are very much correlated with color differences according to human perception. They slightly differ because of the different approaches to their formulation. Nevertheless, both spaces are equally good in perceptual uniformity and provide very good estimates of color difference (distance) between two color vectors [28]. The following steps show the scheme proposed.

- *Selection of a Small Region in the Burn Wound by the user and Preprocessing of the image*. The burn wound will be segmented using the color information of

Fig. 4 Segmentation results:
(**a**) Original image,
(**b**) Segmentation based on
angular distances applied to
hue, (**c**) Segmentation based
on color distances

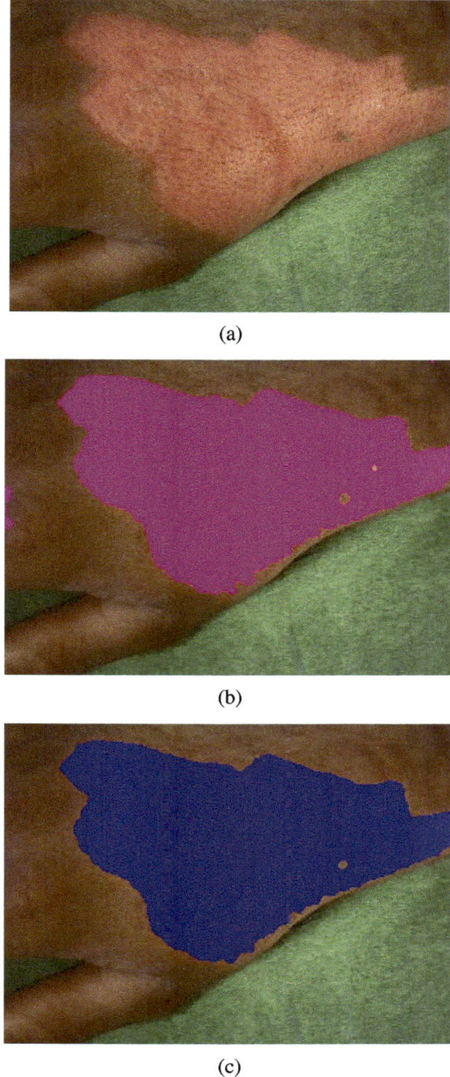

(a)

(b)

(c)

a 5 × 5 pixel area around the point that the user selects with the mouse. Before segmenting the image, it is convenient to preprocess it in order to get more homogeneous regions eliminating noise and small structures. To perform this task, an anisotropic diffusion is applied to the color image [21, 26]. The aim of the diffusion is to make the regions more homogeneous but preserving the edge information. In order to perform the anisotropic diffusion, the approach of separating the diffusion of the chromatic and achromatic information was followed [21].

Fig. 5 Segmentation results:
(**a**) Original image,
(**b**) Segmentation based on
angular distances applied to
hue, (**c**) Segmentation based
on color distances

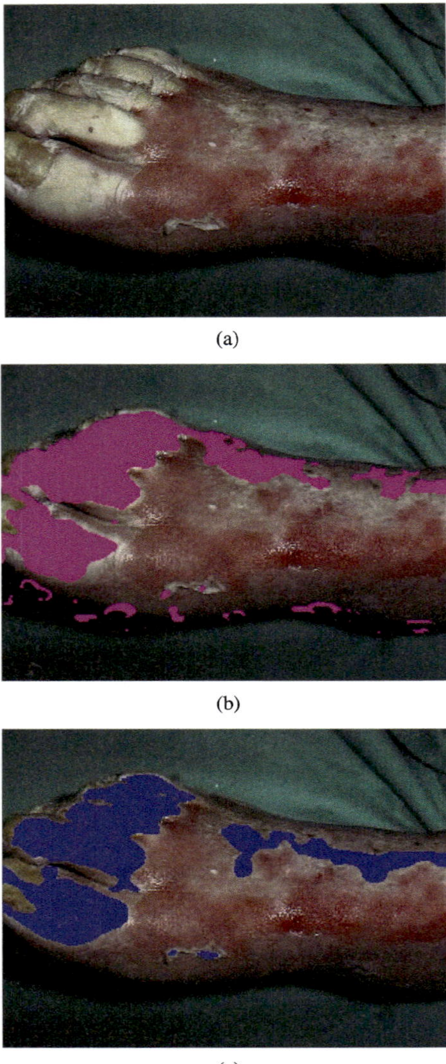

- *Conversion to Single Channel Image.* In this step a single channel image is obtained from the diffused color image. In this gray scale image, differences between the burnt skin selected by the user and other parts of the image are emphasized. Based on the observation that doctors segment burn wounds by measuring differences among colors, the selection box selected by the user is slid as a mask of size 5×5 pixels along the image and, for each pixel in the image under the center of the sliding mask, the following operation is performed:

$$f(m,n) = \frac{1}{MAX} \sum_{i=-\Delta}^{\Delta} \sum_{j=-\Delta}^{\Delta} d_E\big[\mathbf{p}(i+m, j+n),\ \mathbf{w}(i,j)\big], \tag{4}$$

where

$$MAX = \max_{m,n}\left\{ \sum_{i=-\Delta}^{\Delta} \sum_{j=-\Delta}^{\Delta} d_E\big[\mathbf{p}(i+m, j+n),\ \mathbf{w}(i,j)\big] \right\}; \tag{5}$$

$\Delta = (L-1)/2$ with $L=5$; $\mathbf{p}(m,n) = [L_p^*(m,n), u_p^*(m,n), v_p^*(m,n)]^T$ represents a pixel in the filtered image to be segmented in the $L^*u^*v^*$ color space; $\mathbf{w}(i,j) = [L_w^*(i,j), u_w^*(i,j), v_w^*(i,j)]^T$ is a pixel of the mask selected by the user; and $d_E[\ ]$ is the Euclidean distance between the pixels given in the argument. The result of the preceding step is a grayscale image where pixels with the lowest values are those in the region to be segmented. This step has been designed to emphasize the burned regions, and a thresholding operation should suffice to obtain a good segmentation of the wound. The histogram of the distance image is typically multimodal; thus, an optimal threshold to select the mode on the left-hand side or lower-valued side of the histogram needs to be found. This task is carried out in two steps:

1. The peaks (maximum values) of the various modes present in the histogram are found by applying the procedure described in [3].
2. The threshold that separates the two modes close to the lower end of the histogram is calculated by applying Otsu's thresholding method [25].

Finally, a 3×3 median filter is applied to remove spurious pixels in the result of segmentation. The segmentation algorithm described above was tested with 35 burn images, which were also manually segmented by five physicians [37]. The reference image (gold standard) to verify the result of segmentation was obtained by applying a voting method to the regions segmented by the five specialists for each case: a pixel was considered to belong to the segmented (wound) region in the reference image if the majority (at least three) of the physicians had marked it as such. Two parameters were computed to characterize the performance of the segmentation algorithm. The first parameter was the positive predictive value (PPV), which is the ratio between the number of pixels segmented by the algorithm that agree with the reference image and the total number of pixels segmented. The second parameter was the sensitivity, which is the ratio of the number of pixels segmented by the algorithm that agree with the reference image to the total number of pixels marked as wound in the reference image. The first parameter readily characterizes oversegmentation, which would be null if PPV $= 1$; on the other hand, sensitivity gives an indication of undersegmentation. For the 35 images tested in the work of Acha et al. [37], an average sensitivity of 0.8301 was obtained with a standard deviation of 0.09, and an average PPV of 0.9023 was obtained with a standard deviation of 0.078.

3.3 Fuzzy Clustering Algorithms

Castro et al. in [9] present the results of the evaluation of various fuzzy clustering algorithms applied to the segmentation of a heterogeneous set of burn wounds images. The study compares recent and classical algorithms in order to establish a better comparison between the benefits of more complex techniques for pixel classification. RUMA (Relative Ultimate Measurement Accuracy) [42] and a measurement for the global success rate [6] were used to evaluate the success rate of these fuzzy clustering algorithms. The authors conclude that the best algorithm is FKCM (Fuzzy Kernel C-Means) [41], thanks to its excellent results and high stability. However, if it were possible to control the condition in which the photograph is taken, the best algorithm would be MFCM (Modified Fuzzy C-Means) [20]. Both algorithms explained bellow.

3.3.1 Fuzzy Kernel C-Means (FKCM)

This algorithm was proposed by Wu et al. [41]. Before clustering, original data are mapped into a higher dimensional feature space in a nonlinear manner so that each class possess most dissimilarity from other classes. A kernel function is used to make it practical. The R, G, B components of the burn wounds image are the original feature space in [9].

In the following, the image of a input data X_i, $i = 1, 2, \ldots, N$ in the high dimensional feature space is denoted by $\phi(X_i)$, $j = 1, 2, \ldots, M$, where $\phi(\cdot)$ is nonlinear mapping function: $\phi : \mathbf{R}^p \to \mathbf{R}^q$, $p \ll q$. Typical kernel functions are polynomials $K(\mathbf{X}, \mathbf{Y}) = \phi(\mathbf{X}) \cdot \phi(\mathbf{Y}) = (\mathbf{X} \cdot \mathbf{Y} + b)^d$ and radial basis functions $K(\mathbf{X}, \mathbf{Y}) = \phi(\mathbf{X}) \cdot \phi(\mathbf{Y}) = \exp(-(\mathbf{X} - \mathbf{Y})^2 / 2\sigma^2)$. The Euclidean distance between X_i and X_j in the feature space of the kernel K can be defined:

$$d_{ij} = dist\big(\phi(X_i), \phi(X_j)\big) = \sqrt{\left\| \phi(X_i) - \phi(X_j) \right\|^2} \tag{6}$$

and distances can be computed directly from kernel function:

$$d_{ij} = \sqrt{\phi(X_i) \cdot \phi(X_i) - 2\phi(X_i) \cdot \phi(X_j) + \phi(X_j) \cdot \phi(X_j)}$$

$$= \sqrt{K(X_i, X_i) - 2K(X_i, X_j) + K(X_j, X_j)} \tag{7}$$

Based on the original FCM [18], the FKCM algorithm in the high dimensional feature space is as follows:

1. Choose the number of centroids C
2. Choose kernel function K and its parameters
3. Initialize centroids V_j, $j = 1, 2, \ldots, C$
4. Compute the degree of memberships of all feature vectors in all the clusters (u_{ij}, $j = 1, \ldots, C$; $i = 1, \ldots, N$):

$$u_{ij} = \frac{(1/d^2(\mathbf{X}_i, \mathbf{V}_j))^{1/(m-1)}}{\Sigma_{j=1}^{C}(1/d^2(\mathbf{X}_i, \mathbf{V}_j))^{1/(m-1)}} \tag{8}$$

where $d^2(\mathbf{X}_i, \mathbf{V}_j) = K(\mathbf{X}_i, \mathbf{X}_i) - 2K(\mathbf{X}_i, \mathbf{V}_j) + K(\mathbf{V}_j, \mathbf{V}_j)$ and $m \in (1, \infty)$ is a fuzzy index which determines the fuzziness of the clusters.

5. Compute new kernel matrix $K(\mathbf{X}_i, \hat{\mathbf{V}}_j)$ and $K(\hat{\mathbf{V}}_j, \hat{\mathbf{V}}_j)$:

$$K(\mathbf{X}_i, \hat{\mathbf{V}}_j) = \frac{\Sigma_{k=1}^{N}(u_{jk})^m K(\mathbf{X}_k, \mathbf{X}_i)}{\Sigma_{k=1}^{N}(u_{jk})^m} \tag{9}$$

$$K(\hat{\mathbf{V}}_j, \hat{\mathbf{V}}_j) = \frac{\Sigma_{k=1}^{N}\Sigma_{l=1}^{N}(u_{jk})^m (u_{jl})^m K(\mathbf{X}_k, \mathbf{X}_l)}{(\Sigma_{k=1}^{N}(u_{jk})^m)^2} \tag{10}$$

Update the degree of membership u_{ji} to $\hat{u}_{ji}$ according to 8

6. If $\max_{j,i} |u_{ji} - \hat{u}_{ji}| < \varepsilon$ stop, otherwise, go to step 5, where $\varepsilon \in (0, 1)$ is a termination criterion.

3.3.2 Modified Fuzzy C-Means (MFCM)

This algorithm is based on the work of Lim and Lee [20], who describe an algorithm for the segmentation of color images considered as a kind of coarse to fine technique. The coarse segmentation stage attempts to segment coarsely by using the thresholding technique. The histograms of each color band are smoothed by applying scale-space filtering to obtain a set of cut threshold that isolate the color intensity levels appear in the image. The number of regions corresponds to the number of significant peaks in the histogram. The valleys of the histograms correspond to ambiguous areas. The pixels belonging to these areas cannot be assigned to any valid class. These pixels which are not segmented by a coarse segmentation are further segmented using the FCM in the fine segmentation stage.

4 Determination of Burn Depths

Once the burn wound is segmented, the next step is to determine its depth. There are three main types of burn depth [10]:

1. *Superficial dermal burn.* The epidermis and part of the dermis are destroyed. It is characterized by the presence of blisters (usually brown color) and/or a bright red color.
2. *Deep dermal burn.* Its pink-whitish color characterizes it.
3. *Full-thickness burn.* All the skin thickness is destroyed and skin grafts are needed. It is characterized by a beige-yellow or a dark brown color. So, there are five different aspects of the burn wound, although only three depths.

Although a burn wound is classified in three classes, it can present five different appearances.

1. Blisters: they are superficial dermal burns with a bright texture and a rose-brown color.

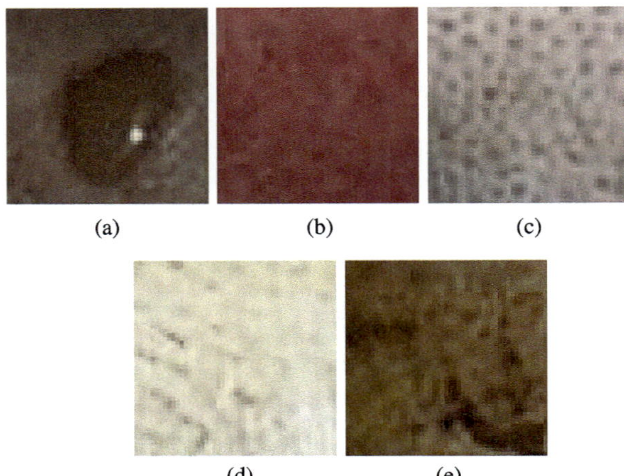

Fig. 6 Different appearances that could present a burn, (**a**) Superficial dermal (*blisters*), (**b**) Superficial dermal (*red*), (**c**) Deep dermal, (**d**) Full thickness (*beige*), (**e**) Full thickness (*brown*)

2. Bright red: they are superficial dermal burns with bright red colors and wet appearance.
3. Pink-white: they are deep dermal burns with a dotted appearance.
4. Yellow-beige: first appearance of full-thickness burns.
5. Brown: second appearance of full-thickness burns.

Examples of each appearance are shown in Fig. 6.

It has been proven that physicians determine the depth of a burn based on color perception, as well as on some texture aspects. In their work, Acha et al. [3] choose features based on a perceptually uniform color space to attain the goal of classifying burn wounds. Fondon et al. [15] try to analyze which features physicians unconsciously take into account to determine the depth and try to translate them into a mathematical quantities. Processes of feature selection have also been addressed in the literature. In [2] a comparison of feature selection results when different classifiers are used, is presented. These issues will be described in this section.

4.1 Features Extraction

4.1.1 Features Based on Color and Statistical Moments

As it has been said, physicians determine the depth of a burn based on color perception and on some texture aspects. In two different studies, two set of color and texture features have been proposed.

In [3], a set of descriptors formed by statistical moments of the histograms obtained for each coordinate of the L*u*v* color space, as well as for the hue and chroma image planes derived from them, were used. L*u*v* space is a perceptually uniform color representation system. Also, the hue and the chroma coordinates are intimately related to the way human beings perceive chromaticity. More specifically, the descriptors chosen were: mean of lightness (L*), mean of hue (h), mean of chroma (c), standard deviation of lightness (σ_L), standard deviation of hue (σ_h), standard deviation of chroma (σ_c), mean of u*, mean of v*, standard deviation of u* (σ_u), standard deviation of v* (σ_v), skewness of lightness (s_L), kurtosis of lightness (k_L), skewness of u* (s_u), kurtosis of u* (k_u), skewness of v* (s_v) and kurtosis of v*. Afterwards it was necessary to apply a descriptor selection method to obtain the optimum set for the subsequent classification.

In the second set of features, coordinates of the L*a*b* color space, the hue and chroma image planes derived from them and RGB coordinates are used. The descriptors chosen in this case are: mean, standard deviation, skewness and kurtosis of red component (R), green component (G) and blue component (B), lightness (L*), a* component (a*), b* component (b*), chroma (C), saturation (S), difference between red band and green band (RG) and difference between blue band and green band (BG). As in the previous features set a feature selection step is needed to analyse the discrimination power of these 40 features.

In Sect. 4.3.3 the results for the feature selection step of these two sets are presented.

4.1.2 Features Extracted from Multidimensional Scaling

Fondon et al. in 2006 [15] proposed to find features which expressed in quantitative measures the experience that physicians use to diagnose and which were closely related to human perception and mathematically well supported. Instead of trying to guess which were the most powerful characteristics in a burn, the authors needed to discover which were the features that consciously or unconsciously were used by the medical experts when they made an assessment.

An experiment was performed with the help of 8 experts and following the Recommendation ITU-R BT. 500-10. A comparison between a pair of images that the medical experts had to rate between 0 and 10, where 0 meant that the images were totally different and 10 that the images ere totally similar was performed. The results were processed with Multidimensional Scaling (MDS) and interpreted with the help of a Hierarchical Cluster Analysis (HCA). The images were projected into the three obtained main dimensions. This graphic was presented to a panel of six experts in Image Processing to identify each dimension with a feature or subjective meaning. The dimension 1 was identified with *amount of pink in the image*, the dimension 2 with *texture of the color* and the dimension 3 with *freshness of the skin*. A further step would be to mathematically describe these subjective characteristics.

4.2 Feature Selection

The discrimination power of the features based on color and statistical moments was analyzed in [3] using the Sequential Forward Selection (SFS) method and the

Sequential Backward Selection (SBS) method [16] via the Fuzzy-ARTMAP neural network which is detailed in the following subsection. Feature selection is to select the best subset from the input space.

SFS is a bottom-up search procedure where one feature at a time is added to the current feature set. At each stage, the feature to be included in the feature set is selected among the remaining available features which have not been added to the feature set. So the new enlarged feature set yields a minimum classification error comparing to adding any single feature. The algorithm stops when adding a new feature yields an increase of the classification error.

The SBS is the top-down counterpart of the SFS method. It starts from the complete set of features and, at each stage, the feature which shows the least discriminatory power is discarded. The algorithm stops when removing another feature implies an increase of the classification error.

To apply these two methods, fifty 49×49 pixel images per each appearance were used. As there are five appearances, there are 250 49×49 pixel images in all.[1] The selection performance was evaluated by fivefold cross validation (XVAL) [17]. In this sense, the disadvantage of sensitiveness to the order of presentation of the training set, that the SBS and SFS methods present, was diminished. To perform the XVAL method the 50 images per burn appearance were split into five disjoint subsets. Four of these subsets (that is, 40 images per appearance) served as training set for the neural network, while the other one (10 images) was used as validation set. Then, the procedure was repeated interchanging the validation subset with one of the training subsets, and so on till the five subsets were used as validation sets. The final classification error was calculated as the mean of the errors for each XVAL run.

4.3 Classifiers Used

The feature selection, explained in the previous section, needs to have an associated classifier. As it has been explained previously, Acha et. al. in [3] used a Fuzzy-ARTMAP neural network as classifier. In a later work [2], the authors made a comparison between that classifier and a non-linear support vector machines with different kernels.

In this section the results of both methods are presented.

4.3.1 Fuzzy-ARTMAP Neural Network

This type of network is based on the Adaptive Resonance Theory developed by Grossberg and Carpenter [8]. Fuzzy-ARTMAP is a supervised learning classifica-

---

[1] The 250 49×49 pixel images were small images showing each one only one burn appearance (no healthy skin or background). Each 49×49 pixel image was validated by two physicians as belonging to a particular depth.

tion architecture for analog-value input pairs of patterns. Fuzzy-ARTMAP offers the advantages of well-understood theoretical properties, an efficient implementation, clustering properties that are consistent with human perception, and a very fast convergence. It has also a track record of successful use in industrial and medical applications [14]. Other strong points of this type of neural network are the small number of design parameters (the vigilance parameter, $o_a \in [0, 1]$, and the selection parameter, $\alpha > 0$) and that the architecture and initial values are always the same, independent of the application.

4.3.2 Support Vector Machine

Support vector algorithms [7] constitute one of the crucial advances about Computational Learning in the 1990s. They are the final step in a long research way known as Statistical Learning, carried out mainly by Vladimir Vapnik [40]. Support Vector Machines are based in the transformation of the input space into another one of higher dimension (usually infinite) in which the problem can be solved by means of a hyperplane optimal (maximum margin). Vector machine formulation is based in the principle of structural risk minimization, which has been shown better than the principle of empirical risk minimization, which is the one used by many conventional neural networks.

The advantages of SVM can be summarized as:

- The training is a problem of convex quadratic programming. Therefore, there are algorithms computationally efficient and the finding of a global extremum is guaranteed.
- It is less susceptible of overfitting than neural networks.
- It allows to work with non-linear relationships between data (it generates non-linear functions by means of kernels).
- It generalizes well with a few training samples.

4.3.3 Feature Selection Results

As already mentioned above, the SFS and SBS methods (Sect. 4.2) needs to have an associated classifier. In this section the results of applying the feature selection to the sets of features based on color and statistical moments presented in Sect. 4.1.1 are summarized in Tables 2 and 3. The average error is calculated counting the misclassifications and dividing by the total number of images used to validate.

Acha et al. [2] presented the results of the feature set based in L*u*v* color space using the Fuzzy-ARTMAP Neural Network and SVM. For the Fuzzy-ARTMAP Neural Network, the SBS feature set (lightness, hue, standard deviation of the hue component, u* chrominance component, standard deviation of the v* component, skewness of lightness) showed the smaller average classification error. SVM was trained using some different kernels. The minimum classification error was obtained for the SVM with 1 variance Gaussian kernel. This classification error was the same,

Table 2 Results of SFS and SBS methods for features based on L*u*v* color space

Classifier	Method	Feature set	Average error
Fuzzy-ARTMAP	SFS	L^*, H, σ_C, u^*, v^*, σ_v, s_L	2 %
	SBS	L^*, H, σ_H, u^*, σ_v, s_L	1.6 %
SVM	SFS	L^*, H, S, σ_S, u^*, σ_{u^*}, s_L	0.7 %

Table 3 Results of SFS for features based on L*a*b* and RGB color spaces

Classifier	Method	Feature set	Average error
Fuzzy-ARTMAP	SFS	a^*, B, σ_{b^*}, S, s_R, R-B, σ_{a^*},	2.1 %

0.7 %, when was used both the SBS and SFS methods. But in the case of SFS method less features were needed, so that was the method chosen. More specifically, 7 features were required. These 7 features were: lightness mean, hue mean, saturation mean, saturation standard deviation, u* mean, u* standard deviation, lightness skewness.

The features set based on L*a*b* color space and RGB components was analysed using only the Fuzzy-ARTMAP neural network as classifier. A 2.1 % classification error was obtained both in SFS and in SBS, however in the case of SFS method the number of features was smaller.

4.4 Classification Results

The features selection allows to obtain the most discriminant features to distinguish between the different depths of burn. These features are used as input to the classifier to characterize images with unknown burn depth.

Acha et al. [3] presented the classification results for the Fuzzy-ARTMAP neural network using the set of selected features based on L*u*v* color space (see Sect. 4.3.3). To test the classification part the authors used 62 images. The neural network was trained with the 250 49 × 49 pixel images previously cited in Sect. 4.2. The training was performed with $\rho_a = 1$ and $\alpha = 0.001$. At the end of the training the weights were fixed for the subsequent classification test. For this test the six features were extracted from the segmented part of the 62 images. The mean value of the 6 features was assigned to each image. Classification results are summarized in Table 4. 22 images with superficial dermal burns, 18 with deep dermal burns and 22 with full-thickness burns were used. The average success percentage was 82.26 %. All superficial dermal burns misclassified were classified by the network as deep dermal ones. All deep dermal burns misclassified were classified by the neural network as superficial dermal ones. And, in the case of misclassified full-thickness burns, 80 % of them were classified as superficial dermal and 20 % as deep dermal.

Table 4 Classification results for the Fuzzy-ARTMAP neural network using the features based on L*u*v*

Burn depth	Success percentage
Superficial dermal	86.36 %
Deep dermal	83.33 %
Full thickness	77.27 %
Average	82.26 %

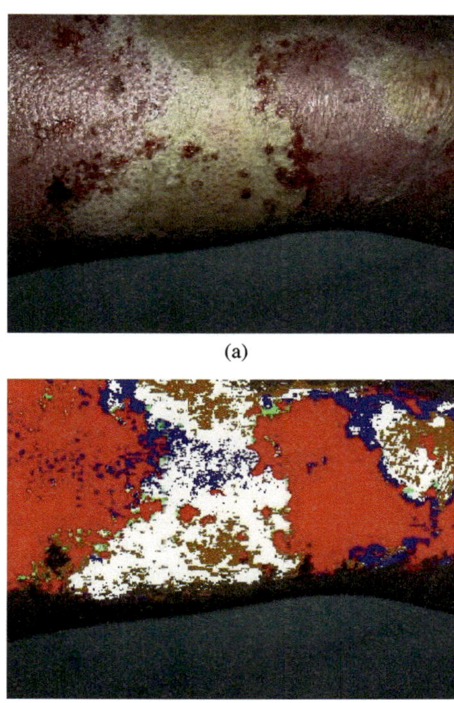

Fig. 7 (**a**) Original image of burn wound. (**b**) Classified lesion, *green* = Superficial dermal (*blisters*), *red* = superficial dermal (*red*), *blue* = deep dermal, *white* = Full thickness (*beige*), *brown* = Full thickness (*brown*)

(a)

(b)

Later, in another analysis, the selected features based on L*a*b* and RGB coordinates have been used as input of the neural network. In this analysis, the network classified each pixel of segmented burn instead of providing an only classification value for the complete segmented burn wound. This yield a pixel-based classification which is very useful since in each image different burn depth can appeared. An example image is shown in Fig. 7 where it can be seen the classification of each pixel individually.

5 Discussion

In this chapter, different efforts existing in the literature to develop a CAD tool for the classification of burns into their depth have been described. Different acquisition methods have been proposed. In this chapter, all the image processing procedures to classify images acquired with digital color camera are described. First, existing method to make color of the burn independent from the acquisition conditions is exposed. Secondly, different methods proposed in the literature to segment the burn are presented. Finally, different color and texture features and different classifiers are utilized to classify. Some methods described in this chapter have been previously published and some others are still unpublished.

References

1. Acha B (2002) Segmentación y clasificación de imágenes en color. Aplicación al diagnóstico de quemaduras. PhD Thesis. Spain: University of Seville
2. Acha B, Serrano C, Palencia S, Murillo JJ (2004) Classification of burn wounds using support vector machines. Proc SPIE Int Soc Opt Eng 5370:1018–1025
3. Acha B, Serrano C, Acha JI, Roa LM (2005) Segmentation and classification of burn images by color and texture information. J Biomed Opt 10(3):1–11
4. Afromowitz MA, Van Liew GS, Heimbach DM (1997) Clinical evaluation of burn injuries using an optical reflectance technique. IEEE Trans Biomed Eng 34:114–127
5. Afromowitz MA, Callis JB, Heimbach DM, DeSoto LA, Norton MK (1988) Multispectral imaging of burn wounds: a new clinical instrument for evaluating burn depth. IEEE Trans Biomed Eng 35:842–850
6. Alonso Betanzos A, Arcay Varela B, Castro Martinez A (2000) Analysis and evaluation of hard and fuzzy clustering segmentation techniques in burned patient images. Image Vis Comput 18(13):1045–1054
7. Burges CJC (1998) A tutorial on support vector machines for pattern recognition. Data Min Knowl Discov 2:2
8. Carpenter GA, Grossberg S, Markuzon S, Reynolds JH (1992) Fuzzy-ARTMAP: a neural network architecture for incremental supervised learning of analog multidimensional maps. IEEE Trans Neural Netw 5:698–713
9. Castro A, Bóveda C, Arcay B (2006) Analysis of fuzzy clustering algorithms for the segmentation of burn wounds photographs. Lect Notes Comput Sci 4142:491–501
10. Clarke JA (1992) A colour atlas of burn injuries. Chapman & Hall Medical, London
11. Cole RP, Jones SG, Shakespeare PG (1990) Thermographic assessment of hand burns. Burns 16(1):60–63
12. Doi K (2006) Diagnostic imaging over the last 50 years: research and development in medical imaging science and technology. Phys Med Biol 51(13):R5–R27
13. Doi K (2007) Computer-aided diagnosis in medical imaging: historical review, current status and future potential. Comput Med Imaging Graph 31(4–5):198–211
14. Donohoe GW, Nemeth S, Soliz P (1998) ART-based image analysis for pigmented lesions of the skin. In: 11th IEEE symposium on computer-based medical systems, pp 293–298
15. Fondón I, Acha B, Serrano C, Sosa M (2006) New characteristics for the classification of burns: experimental study. Lect Notes Comput Sci 4142:502–512
16. Fukunaga K (1990) Introduction to statistical pattern recognition, 2nd edn. Morgan Kaufmann, San Diego

17. Ganster H, Pinz A, Röhrer R, Wilding E, Binder M, Kittler H (2001) Automated melanoma recognition. IEEE Trans Med Imaging 3:233–239
18. Gath I, Geva AB (1989) Unsupervised optimal fuzzy clustering. IEEE Trans Pattern Anal Mach Intell 11(7):773–780
19. Huang SY, Macpherson E, Zhang YT (2007) A feasibility study of burn wound depth assessment using terahertz pulsed imaging. In: Proceedings of the 4th IEEE-EMBS international summer school and symposium on medical devices and biosensors, ISSS-MDBS 2007, pp 132–135
20. Lim YW, Lee SU (1990) On the color image segmentation algorithm based on the thresholding and the fuzzy c-means techniques. Pattern Recognit 23(9):935–952
21. Lucchese L, Mitra SK (2001) Color segmentation based on separate anisotropic diffusion of chromatic and achromatic channels. IEEE Proc Vis Image Signal Process 148(3):141–150
22. McLaren K (1976) The development of the CIE 1976 (l*a*b*) uniform colourspace and colour-difference formula. J Soc Dyers Colour 92:338–341
23. Monstrey SM, Hoeksema H, Baker RD, Jeng J, Spence RS, Wilson D, Pape SA (2011) Burn wound healing time assessed by laser Doppler imaging. Part 2: validation of a dedicated colour code for image interpretation. Burns 37(2):249–256
24. Niazi ZBM, Essex TJH, Papini R, Scott D, McLean NR, Black JM (1993) New laser Doppler scanner, a valuable adjunct in burn depth assessment. Burns 19(6):485–489
25. Otsu N (1979) A threshold selection method from gray-level histograms. IEEE Trans Syst Man Cybern 9(1):62–66
26. Perona P, Malik J (1990) Scale-space and edge detection using anisotropic diffusion. IEEE Trans Pattern Anal Mach Intell 12(7):629–639
27. Pierce MC, Sheridan RL, Park BH, Cense B, De Boer JF (2003) Burn depth determination in human skin using polarization-sensitive optical coherence tomography. Proc SPIE Int Soc Opt Eng 4956:263–270
28. Plataniotis KN, Venetsanopoulos AN (2000) Color image processing and applications. Springer, Berlin
29. Rangayyan RM (2005) Biomedical image analysis. CRC, Boca Raton
30. Rangayyan RM, Acha B, Serrano C (2011) Color image processing with biomedical applications. SPIE press monograph, vol PM206
31. Renkielska A, Nowakowski A, Kaczmarek M, Ruminski J (2006) Burn depths evaluation based on active dynamic IR thermal imaging-A preliminary study. Burns 32(7):867–875
32. Roa L, Gómez-Cía T, Acha B, Serrano C (1999) Digital imaging in remote diagnosis of burns. Burns 25(7):617–623
33. Romero-Méndez R, Jiménez-Lozano JN, Sen M, Javier González F (2009) Analytical solution of the Pennes equation for burn-depth determination from infrared thermographs. Math Med Biol 27(1):21–38
34. Ruminski J, Kaczmarek M, Renkielska A, Nowakowski A (2007) Thermal parametric imaging in the evaluation of skin burn depth. IEEE Trans Biomed Eng 54(2):303–312. Art. no. 14
35. Sáez A, Acha B, Serrano C (2009) Colorimetric calibration of images captured under unknown illuminants. In: Proceedings of the 11th congress of the international colour association (Aic), Sidney, Australia
36. Serrano C, Roa L, Acha B (1998) Evaluation of a telemedicine platform in a burn unit. In: Proceedings of the IEEE international conference on information technology applications in biomedicine, Washington, DC, pp 121–126
37. Serrano C, Acha B, Gómez-Cía T, Acha JI, Roa LM (2005) A computer assisted diagnosis tool for the classification of burns by depth of injury. Burns 31(3):275–281
38. Serrano C, Acha B, Sangwine SJ (2005) Colorimetric calibration of images of human skin captured under hospital conditions. In: Proceedings of the 10th congress of the international colour association AIC, Granada, Spain, vol 1, pp 773–776
39. Tannenbaum B (2007) Webinar color image processing with MATLAB. June 28th
40. Vapnik V (1995) The nature of statistical learning theory. Springer, New York

41. Wu Z, Xie W, Yu J (2003) Fuzzy C-means clustering algorithm based on kernel method. In: Computational intelligence and multimedia applications, ICCIMA, pp 49–54
42. Zhang YJ (1996) A survey on evaluation methods for image segmentation. Pattern Recognit 29(8):1335–1346

Index

M.E. Celebi, G. Schaefer (eds.), *Color Medical Image Analysis*, 203
Lecture Notes in Computational Vision and Biomechanics 6,
DOI 10.1007/978-94-007-5389-1, © Springer Science+Business Media Dordrecht 2013